HEAL WITH
DETOX

Dr Ho See Yunn

About this book

Heal With Detox explains detoxification in a nutshell. It is dedicated to patients to achieve a cure for their chronic ailments by eliminating toxins, which is a significant root cause of diseases. This book gathers evidence-based approaches from functional medicine and swiss biological medicine perspectives. It summarizes why we need to detox in today's world, the principles of testing and diagnosis for heavy metals and how to enhance your body's own detoxification for healing. If you have been trying to seek healing for your condition but have been going in circles trying to find a cause, then this book is for you.

Heal With Detox is a practical guide for patients who want to understand more about toxicity in our environment and how to properly diagnose it or even assess the level of toxicity the patient may be at. Suppose you are suffering from chronic gut conditions like Irritable Bowel Syndrome, neurodegenerative brain disorders like Parkinson's and Alzheimer's, Multiple Chemical Sensitivity, skin conditions like Psoriasis or chronic allergies, or even metabolic or cardiovascular conditions, then this book will be a stepping stone to help achieve greater healing if you are at a standstill in your healing journey.

This book also comes with tips on detoxifying even at home with nutritional principles and detoxification recipes you can use at home to alkalinize your body and enhance the liver's detoxification process.

About the Author

Dr Ho See Yunn is a Family Physician with over 15 years' experience. Dr Ho holds a diploma from the New York Institute of Integrative Medicine in Integrative Health and Nutrition. She received her Advanced Fellowship in Functional and Nutritional medicine and peptide certification from the American Academy of Anti-ageing and Regenerative Medicine. Also, Dr Ho received biological medicine training in the Swiss Biological Medicine Academy. Dr Ho is also trained and certified under Dr. Walsh's advanced nutrient therapy protocols that use personalized nutrient treatment strategies to treat mood and behavioral disorders. Dr Ho believes in treating the patient holistically and finding the underlying root causes of disease. She takes a biochemical, nutritional and genetic approach in managing patients with chronic diseases.

"I have written this book with the hope that the content of this book will allow patients and practitioners to have a deeper understanding of the various sources of toxins in our environment and how it affects our body to cause illness, how to assess your level of toxicity and what are the various options now to test for toxicity. There are also tips on the various methods of detoxification to help your body develop its own natural healing."

Preface and Disclaimer

This book was written as detoxification is still a much untouched upon topic between practitioners and patients. I wanted to increase the awareness of how detoxification can be the first step to achieving more optimal health after seeing many patients benefit from it.

Our environment is becoming more toxic every day and never in human history have we been inundated with such high numbers of toxin-related illnesses and immune attacking viruses.

Detoxification is a rapidly emerging field of medicine. It only is touched upon by occupational medicine doctors as patients usually get toxin related illnesses from their workplace. I have recently seen toxin-related illnesses presenting everywhere. More toxins like lead and mercury leaks into our waters and food chains and end up in the human body, triggering our immune system to be overactive and causing rising cases of diseases like Hashimoto's disease or rising infertility.

There has been much controversy surrounding detoxification also since there is not much scientific certainty about this topic. However, throughout the years, many doctors or naturopaths have been practicing detoxification to heal diseases and have achieved good patient outcomes, although they have not been published as scientific data to be recognized by the scientific community. Many holistic doctors on the frontlines have realized the epidemic portion of toxicity-related illnesses and are trying to help patients with their diagnosis and treatment using detoxification. Hopefully, over time, there will be more research and scientific data emerging from this field to resolve its controversies.

As much as I have tried to present the information in this book as accurate as possible, data changes relatively fast and I can only hope to update the information in this book to keep them current. This book is cumulated from hours of research but is still a work in progress and cannot be a diagnostic or treatment manual. Though every effort has been made to ensure the accuracy of this book's information, it is not meant to provide medical advice as that can only come from your own treating physician. The material in this book is not intended to be a substitute for proper medical advice from one's own physician or other healthcare providers. It simply reflects the latest thoughts and trends in this field and from my own personal experiences. I would also like to put a disclaimer I have no financial ties to any supplement or pharmaceutical company or laboratory in writing this book. The author of this book shall not be liable for any loss, injury, or damage arising from any information in this book.

Acknowledgements

I would like to thank God for guiding me to be at a unique position where I am – not just a conventional trained doctor, but also a doctor that has been trained in Functional Medicine and in the Swiss biological method of healing. I would also like to thank my parents for being always supportive of me and enabling me to always pursue my dreams to be a doctor since I was a child. I am forever grateful to my mum and dad for teaching me the bible and I dedicate this book to my dad whose medical condition led me into functional medicine to treat patients from the root cause of their problems.

Last but not least, I would like to thank my husband Terry for always encouraging me to pursue my passion in Functional medicine and getting my training and certification despite having to juggle my role as a busy clinician and a mum of two. He is always supportive of me to continue studying and helping to take care of the family while I continue to pursue my passion. This book would not see its light without my husband constantly encouraging me.

Content Page

CHAPTER 1

Introduction

While it was once rare to develop sensitivities to multiple environmental triggers, it is becoming more and more common. A growing number of physicians are seeing more "difficult to treat" sensitive patients due to the significant increase in toxins in our world. Every day, we are exposed to a myriad of chemicals that were non-existent fifty years ago. These include organic pollutants, heavy metals, and even electromagnetic radiation through the products we use on our bodies and electronics we hold near our brains all day long. To make the scenario more dire, the multiple chemical disasters like the Fukushima nuclear accident has caused more harmful chemicals to be emitted into the air we breathe, the waters we drink, and the food chain. We are being exposed to an unprecedented amount of highly toxic chemicals and radiation and there has been little awareness or studies into what impact this has on our bodies. (1)

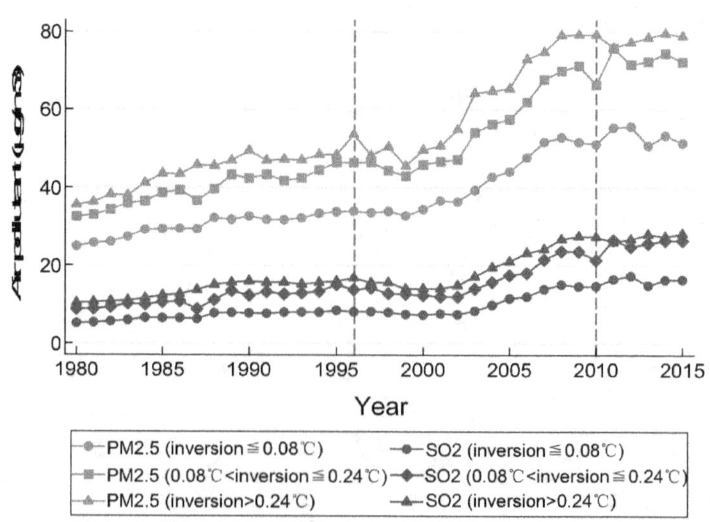

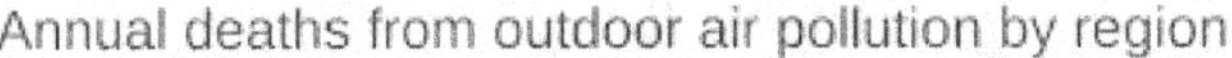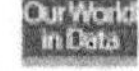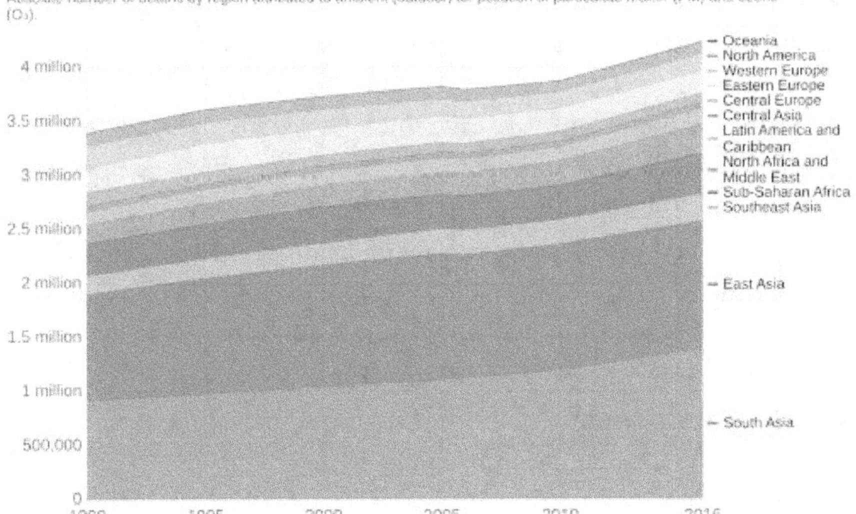

Global air quality has been deteriorating since 1990, with an approximate 1.2% increase overall in the last 15 years. Air quality, specifically particulate matter in the air, has also been ranked as the 5th leading cause of death worldwide, alongside factors such as smoking, diet and high blood pressure, and has been estimated to cause about 4.2 million deaths annually. (2)

All these toxicities are challenging our body's immune system and triggering an unseen precedent of autoimmunity and sensitivity reactions. In recent years, there has been an epidemic increase in chronic fatigue syndrome, fibromyalgia, multiple chemical sensitive rises, cancer, mould toxicity, and neurodegenerative disease.

To paint a more realistic picture of the severity, the prevalence of multiple chemical sensitivity (MCS) is noted in recent research to involve 3.2 percent of the US population, roughly 10 million people!

Why do some people survive well in this environment while some people succumb to years of suffering from toxicity and sensitivity? This boils down to genetic susceptibility and also the amount of exposure that accumulates in the body beyond the body's ability to detoxify and excrete them.

The period of working with these "chronically sick" patients who have suffered for many years may take from six months to five years or more. It takes patience and perseverance to heal these patients who have been suffering from so many years of pain and fatigue.

Heavy metal toxicity causes chronic cellular dysfunctions, thus contributing to many diseases. In a biological sense, they often cause blockages in a cell's reactive capability. They act on various organs and can present as disorders in multiple systems, especially the weakened ones. Heavy metal intoxication can remain sub-clinically dormant until the weakening of the body brings the toxicity to present clinically.

Manifestations of heavy metal toxicity

1) Mucosal symptoms
- asthma or recurrent bronchitis
- sinusitis
- recurring stomatitis, ulcers
- colitis
- recurring cystitis, vaginitis

2) Neurological symptoms
- recurrent headaches, migraine
- brain fog
- trigeminal nerve pain
- vertigo
- mood disorders
- muscle weakness
- chronic fatigue
- tremors
- chronic insomnia

3) Skin
- hair loss
- eczema
- recurrent urticaria / hives

Heavy metal intoxication should not be treated individually, but rather must be given constitutional treatment as well. For example, copper is normally stored in the liver and is a mediator of reactivity and inflammability. Copper intoxication results in increased inflammation in the body or even autoimmunity. In TCM, it is called the Yang and corresponds to rage, anger and heat. It is important when treating high copper to work on the liver and bile elimination and providing an avenue to work off energy (i.e., cell respiration with elemental iron). This is the constitutional treatment of chronic inflammation, which usually presents with high copper and low zinc. These constitutional problems usually would not resolve unless the heavy metals are eliminated.

Heavy metal intoxication is only one part of the "disease manifestation" and usually manifests with other intoxications. For example, just removing amalgam from a root canal treated tooth cannot solve the problem and sometimes may even trigger stronger symptoms as it shifts the toxic cadaverous proteins in the root into the mesenchymal tissues. A good biological dentist would look to remove the filling with the dead tooth and the cadaverous bone associated with it.

The aim of this book is to bring awareness about the effects of toxins on our body and what we can do to find a diagnosis and treatment if toxicity is affecting you or your family member's health. I have seen many patients lost in the complexities of the medical system trying to find an answer for their health issues and often being told that "it is just in your head" or given a diagnosis of "chronic fatigue" or "irritable bowel syndrome" without an end in sight for their many years of suffering. The aim of this book is to provide a compass for patients to begin the journey of healing by understanding firstly how toxicity can be an important underlying cause of their health problems and how they can find help to diagnose and treat the health conditions they have been suffering from. We will dig further into how toxicity can manifest as illnesses in different organ systems and help guide patients to consider therapeutic intervention to remove toxins from the body, especially in chronically ill patients who are not responding to conventional therapeutic interventions. This book also provides insights into how daily detoxification strategies can be incorporated into our daily habits, and ending off with detoxification recipes to help with our own body's detoxification.

The "3 pillar" approach is useful to help achieve optimal health. First is to cleanse the body of toxins. Second, we work to balance the gut health and third, we help the cells in our body to regenerate and repair. In recent years, the increasing level of toxicity in our environment and viral epidemic has brought a growing trend of patients who are sicker and presenting with more vague symptoms than before. These patients usually present with unexplained fatigue, pain, brain fog or cognitive decline, mood issues like depression and anxiety and extreme allergies or sensitivities to their environment. Some of these patients are also extremely sensitive to any supplements or medications given until the body is first cleared of toxins and the gut is rebalanced.

The approach to detoxification starts with working on the patient's diet and lifestyle to reduce toxic exposure and to work at finding underlying causes for the symptoms that the patients are experiencing. There is an extensive panel of functional tests to help in the diagnosis of toxicity from serum acute toxicity blood tests to urine heavy metals challenge tests to diagnose chronic toxicity. There are also tests to check for organic pollutant toxicity and mold toxicity. In addition, genetic susceptibility causing poor detoxification can be investigated by looking at detoxification genetic SNPs, which could predispose the patient to more toxic effects from the environment. A much-neglected source of toxins is also dental toxins. It is also important to work closely with a biological dentist to safely remove dental sources of toxicity, for example, mercury amalgams and root canals, so that patients have better outcomes when they embark on detoxification to heal their body.

CHAPTER 2

How toxic are you: assessing your level of toxicity

Toxicity can manifest in our body in both acute or chronic ways. Many of today's chronic illnesses are due to the multiple toxic exposures we accumulate from our environment.

Toxicity can manifest as acute symptoms that appear immediately after exposure. But it can also appear as chronic vague symptoms that manifest after many years of exposure and accumulation in our bodies. Soon these toxin exposures overwhelm our body's own detoxification ability and cause symptoms including:

- Fatigue
- Chronic headaches
- Body pains and aches
- Sleep issues
- Headaches

Many of these symptoms are left unnoticed or even dismissed by physicians, but if allowed to accumulate without treating the toxicity, it can lead to:

- cardiovascular disease
- autoimmune disease
- cancer
- neurodegenerative diseases

Sadly, in medicine nowadays, doctors usually treat the symptoms without looking at the underlying causes of diseases. When skin rashes appear, steroid creams are used to suppress the symptoms. When autoimmune diseases occur, immunosuppressants and steroids are used to suppress our immune system. When neurodegenerative diseases occur, drugs are prescribed to boost dopamine. But these treatments usually make symptoms subside for a while, but if the underlying toxicity is not addressed, the immune system will be activated again as the body's way of coping with the toxin exposure.

A journal review in 2015 Carcinogenesis revealed that even though lifestyle factors cause the majority of cancers, the World Health Organization and the International Agency for Research on Cancer (IARC) suggest that the fraction of cancers attributable to toxic environmental exposures is between 7% and 19%. The study suggested that the cumulative effects of individual (non-carcinogenic) chemicals acting on different pathways, and a variety of related systems, organs, tissues and cells could plausibly conspire to produce carcinogenic synergies.

There are more than a hundred types of environmental toxins that could trigger toxic reactions in our body and overwhelm our detoxification ability. Some of the common ones include:

1. Heavy metals like Arsenic, Cadmium, Lead, Mercury - these can come from the food we eat, the water we drink, the air we breathe, and the products we use daily.

2. Solvents or Volatile Organic Compounds - These can come from cleaning products or anything that emits an odour, for example, newly painted furniture.

3. Pesticides and Glyphosate - these can come from the vegetables we eat.

Assessing your level of toxicity
(Adapted from IFM toxicity questionnaire)
I)   Assessing your level of exposure to toxins

Toxin Exposure Questionnaire (TEQ-20)

Patient Name____ Date_______________

Please check YES or NO for each of the following questions. Your provider will discuss your answers with you.

	QUESTIONS	YES	NO
1.	Do you consume conventionally grown (non-organic) fruits and vegetables regularly? If so, which ones do you eat most often? _____________	☐	☐
2.	Do you consume conventionally raised animal products (meat, dairy, eggs) regularly? If so, which ones do you eat most often? _____________	☐	☐
3.	Do you consume fish or seafood more than twice a week? If so, please describe what you eat and whether it is farmed or wild. _____________	☐	☐
4.	Do you consume fast foods, canned/packaged foods, soda, or foods with artificial colors, flavors, preservatives or sweeteners more than three times a week?	☐	☐
5.	Have you lived in a mobile home, boat, or RV, or a very old or brand-new home? If so, please describe: _____________	☐	☐
6.	Have you recently been exposed to new construction materials or furniture (e.g., paint, laminate flooring, particle board, new carpeting, bedding, furniture, etc.)?	☐	☐
7.	Does your home or workplace have cracking paint or decaying insulation or foam, visible mold, water damage, or damp windows, basement, or crawlspaces?	☐	☐
8.	Are you often exposed to adhesives, paints, flea treatments, varnishes, solvents, welding/soldering materials, or other air-borne chemicals at home or work?	☐	☐
9.	Have you been exposed to treated lumber, lead paint, paint chips or dust, broken mercury thermometers or fluorescent bulbs, or other toxic substances you know of?	☐	☐
10.	Do you drink water from a well, spring, or cistern, or from plumbing pipes or fixtures installed before 1986?	☐	☐
11.	Do you regularly use conventional cleaning chemicals, disinfectants, hand sanitizers, air fresheners, scented candles, or other scented products at home or work?	☐	☐
12.	Are your health concerns related to time spent living or working adjacent to a highway, factory, incinerator, gas station, power plant, or other industrial pollution source?	☐	☐
13.	Have you lived in an agricultural area or often been exposed to herbicides, pesticides, fungicides at home, work, parks & golf courses, or roadsides?	☐	☐
14.	Do you live near a cell phone tower, high-voltage power lines, or other known source of electromagnetic radiation?	☐	☐
15.	Do you live or work in a sealed building with recirculated air or a building that has wood, propane, or gas stoves or appliances?	☐	☐
16.	Do you smoke or are often exposed to second-hand smoke, fly often, or run or bike to work along busy streets?	☐	☐
17.	Are you highly sensitive to smoke, perfumes, fragrances, cleaning products, gasoline, or other fumes? If so, please explain: _____________	☐	☐
18.	Have you had root canals, tooth extractions, "silver" fillings, crowns, dental sealants, dentures, retainers, aligning trays, braces, mouth guards, dental implants, etc.?	☐	☐
19.	Have you had any unusual reactions to anesthesia or to prescription or over-the-counter medications? If so, please describe: _____________	☐	☐
20.	Do you have a history of heavy use of alcohol or recreational or prescription drugs? If so, please describe or discuss with your provider: _____________	☐	☐

II) Assessing your level of toxic symptoms - https://drhyman.com/downloads/MSQ_Fillable.pdf

MSQ - MEDICAL SYMPTOM/TOXICITY QUESTIONNAIRE

NAME: ________________________________   **DATE:** ________________

The Toxicity and Symptom Screening Questionnaire identifies symptoms that help to identify the underlying causes of illness, and helps you track your progress over time. Rate each of the following symptoms based upon your health profile for the past 30 days. If you are taking after the first time, record your symptoms for the last 48 hours ONLY.

POINT SCALE

0 = Never or almost never have the symptom
1 = Occasionally have it, effect is not severe
2 = Occasionally have, effect is severe
3 = Frequently have it, effect is not severe
4 = Frequently have it, effect is severe

DIGESTIVE TRACT
____ Nausea or vomiting
____ Diarrhea
____ Constipation
____ Bloated feeling
____ Belching, or passing gas
____ Heartburn
____ Intestinal/Stomach pain
Total **0**

EARS
____ Itchy ears Total
____ Earaches, ear infections
____ Drainage from ear
____ Ringing in ears, hearing loss
Total **0**

EMOTIONS
____ Mood swings
____ Anxiety, fear or nervousness
____ Anger, irritability, or aggressiveness
____ Depression
Total **0**

ENERGY/ACTIVITY
____ Fatigue, sluggishness
____ Apathy, lethargy
____ Hyperactivity
____ Restlessness
Total **0**

EYES
____ Watery or itchy eyes
____ Swollen, reddened or sticky eyelids
____ Bags or dark circles under eyes
____ Blurred or tunnel vision (does not include near-or far-sightedness)
Total **0**

HEAD
____ Headaches
____ Faintness
____ Dizziness
____ Insomnia
Total **0**

HEART
____ Irregular or skipped heartbeat
____ Rapid or pounding heartbeat
____ Chest pain
Total **0**

JOINTS/MUSCLES
____ Pain or aches in joints
____ Arthritis
____ Stiffness or limitation of movement
____ Pain or aches in muscles
____ Feeling of weakness or tiredness
Total **0**

LUNGS
____ Chest congestion
____ Asthma, bronchitis
____ Shortness of breath
____ Difficult breathing
Total **0**

MIND
____ Poor memory
____ Confusion, poor comprehension
____ Poor concentration
____ Poor physical coordination
____ Difficulty in making decisions
____ Stuttering or stammering
____ Slurred speech
____ Learning disabilities
Total **0**

MOUTH/THROAT
____ Chronic coughing
____ Gagging, frequent need to clear throat
____ Sore throat, hoarseness, loss of voice
____ Swollen/discolored tongue, gum, lips
____ Canker sores
Total **0**

NOSE
____ Stuffy nose
____ Sinus problems
____ Hay fever
____ Sneezing attacks
____ Excessive mucus formation
Total **0**

SKIN
____ Acne
____ Hives, rashes, or dry skin
____ Hair loss
____ Flushing or hot flushes
____ Excessive sweating
Total **0**

WEIGHT
____ Binge eating/drinking
____ Craving certain foods
____ Excessive weight
____ Compulsive eating
____ Water retention
____ Underweight
Total **0**

OTHER
____ Frequent illness
____ Frequent or urgent urination
____ Genital itch or discharge
Total **0**

GRAND TOTAL ____ 0

KEY TO QUESTIONNAIRE
Add individual scores and total each group. Add each group scores and give a grand total.
• Optimal is less than 10   • Mild Toxicity: 10-50   • Moderate Toxicity: 50-100   • Severe Toxicity: over 100

Heavy metals can be tested through a blood or urine sample to determine if you have been exposed to these metals in your environment. Blood tests may reveal recent exposure as blood cells turnover within 3-4 months. A Urine Heavy Metal challenge test can give a better picture of the total body burden. The heavy metals panel usually checks for mercury, lead, cadmium, aluminum and arsenic.

There are many different tests in the market to determine a person's exposure and how much of it is accumulating in the body. The tests also include genetic testing to assess a person's susceptibility to poor detoxification. These tests include:

- Blood heavy metal tests: This indicates current heavy metal exposure as these heavy metals stay in the blood for about ninety days that is the duration of turnover of blood cells. There are also newer blood tests that can distinguish between inorganic mercury exposure (from fillings or pollution) and organic mercury exposure (from fish). However, this test doesn't address heavy metals stored in bones, organs and tissues.

- Hair testing: this is a simple and effective way to determine exposure to heavy metals and also to detect mineral deficiencies in the body as meals remain in the hair for several weeks after exposure. However, opponents will say that the hair analysis is not as accurate as blood and urine tests for determining the heavy metal load in the body. For mercury, the hair analysis is not the appropriate methods for analysis as hair belongs to part of the skin and mercury is hardly ever excreted via the skin, causing false low values. Hair mineral analysis is more sensitive to aluminum and lead.

- Urine chelation challenge test: this test is performed using oral or intravenous chelating agents and checking the urine before and after the provoking challenge. This is the most appropriate test for checking for long term body burden of heavy metals as it pulls out the heavy metals from the body and shows up in the urine.

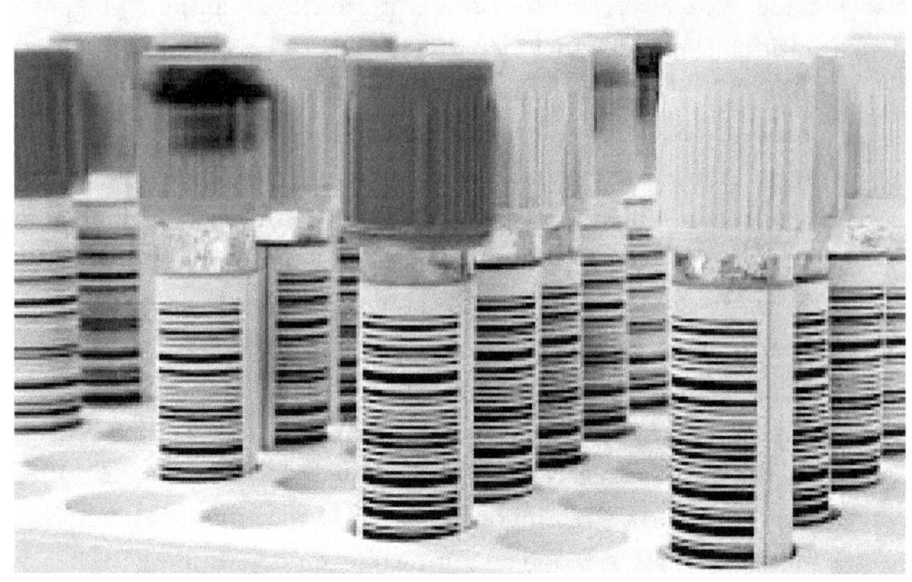

Testing for detoxification capability

Free radicals that accumulate in our bodies can damage our cells and make us susceptible to the toxin-related illnesses. Thankfully, mother nature has equipped our bodies to make antioxidants to turn these harmful free radicals into harmless substances to be excreted from our bodies. Testing for genetic variants in the various antioxidant pathways will help us to determine whether our bodies can make antioxidants for adequate detoxification.

1. The Superoxide Dismutase pathway (SOD)

The antioxidant called Superoxide Dismutase (SOD) takes superoxide and turns it into hydrogen peroxide before the other antioxidants catalase and glutathione breaks the hydrogen peroxide into water and oxygen.

The genes SOD 1, SOD2, and SOD3 are needed to make superoxide dismutase. Genetic variation in the SOD gene will cause disruption in the function and make a person more susceptible to toxins and its health issues.

We can boost SOD naturally from plant products. However, when SOD is ingested in the body, it is quickly destroyed by stomach acids and intestinal enzymes. Fortunately, it is possible to boost levels of this important antioxidant by consuming supplements that supply concentrated amounts of appropriate precursor molecules. Wheat sprouts represent one rich source of these SOD-boosting building blocks, and have been shown to significantly increase internal antioxidant levels. In another study, a French team examined the antioxidant and anti-inflammatory properties of SOD extracted from melon, in both laboratory cell studies and live animals. Their studies showed that the antioxidant properties attributed to the melon extract were indeed due to active SOD. Some studies have shown that polyphenols from apple skins may support SOD production as well. (12)

2. Catalase (CAT)

Catalase is another important enzyme in the antioxidant pathway, which helps convert the hydrogen peroxide into oxygen and water. Variants in the CAT genes may impair your ability to detoxify free radicals. There is hence more hydrogen peroxide to react with iron to form hydroxyl radicals. If you have a high level of iron in your body from supplementation or dietary sources of iron, you will be more susceptible to this Fenton reaction to create free radicals creating harmful effects on the cells.

There is a study by the University of Bradford on the role of enzyme Catalase in the hair greying process. The study that oxidative stress causes the hair follicles to overproduce hydrogen peroxide, which bleaches the hair and makes it grey. (13) Foods that contain natural sources of catalase include beef liver, wheat sprouts, lentils, brussel sprouts and other foods, including cheese, yeast, sunflower seeds and dairy products also contain catalase.

3. Glutathione (GST)

Glutathione is a master antioxidant used by the liver to clear many toxins both in Phase I and phase II detoxification. It helps to protect the body against free radicals and maintain the cell's redox potential. Glutathione levels decline as we age and make the body prone to toxin-related health issues and inflammation. Genetic variants can insufficiently produce glutathione and cause serious detoxification issues. Besides the production of glutathione, it is also important to recycle glutathione from the oxidized form back to the reduced form, so it is available again to grab free radicals in the body. There are blood tests we can do to measure the level of oxidized and reduced glutathione.

You can compensate for low glutathione. The most effective form is liposomal glutathione, which has better absorption in the intestines. Another effective form is S-acetyl glutathione or taking glutathione precursors like N-acetyl-cysteine (NAC).

4. Nrf2 genes

Nrf2 controls enzymes that produce and utilize glutathione to support the antioxidant process to neutralize free radicals. Genetic variants in the Nrf2 gene may impair this process and subject the body to inflammation. Natural sources to boost Nrf2 pathways include sulforaphane from broccoli, resveratrol, milk thistle and turmeric to support a healthy Nrf2 activity.

So do discuss with your functional medicine practitioner your options for heavy metals and genetic testing if you are suffering from health issues like autoimmune disorders, cancer or other toxin-related illnesses to improve detoxification from the genetic and cellular level.

CHAPTER 3

Sources of Heavy Metals

Heavy metals are naturally occurring elements in our environment. However, since the industrial revolution, the multiple and heavy use of heavy metals in industrial, domestic, agricultural, medical and technological industries have led to the widespread distribution of these heavy metals seeping into our environment, entering our food chains and accumulating in our bodies, causing toxic health effects. These heavy metals have entered the air we breathe, the water we drink and the foods we eat at an alarming level due to the effects of environmental pollution.

Some of these heavy metals are required as trace elements in our body, for example, chromium, zinc and copper function as cofactors for enzyme functions. However, the toxicity of these heavy metals depends on the dose of our exposure, the route of exposure, the chemical type, as well as our age, underlying medical issues, genetics and nutritional status to determine their impact on our bodies.

Here, we have highlighted five major metals with a high degree of toxicity - namely lead, mercury, arsenic, cadmium and chromium. These heavy metals, if allowed to accumulate, may have systemic effects on our body, causing damage to multiple organs, even carcinogenesis.

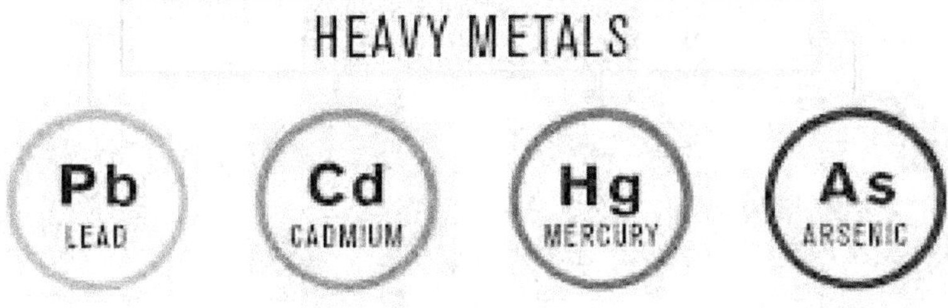

I) Lead

Sources of lead exposure
- Inhalation of lead-contaminated dust particles or aerosols
- Ingestion of lead-contaminated food, water, and paints. Adults absorb 35 to 50% of lead through drinking water and the absorption rate for children may be greater than 50%. (14)
- Contact with lead in deteriorating household paints
- Lead in the workplace
- Lead in crystals and ceramic containers that leach into water and food
- Lead use in hobbies
- Lead use in some traditional medicines and cosmetics
- Water from pipes in old buildings
- Inhalation of exhaust fumes from vehicles

Effects of lead exposure
- The nervous system is the most vulnerable target of lead poisoning. Headache, poor attention span, irritability, loss of memory and dullness are the early symptoms of the effects of lead exposure on the central nervous system. (15)
- In children, studies have shown an association between blood level poisoning and diminished intelligence, lower intelligence quotient-IQ, delayed or impaired neurobehavioral development, decreased hearing acuity, speech and language handicaps, growth retardation, poor attention span, and anti-social and diligent behaviors.
- In the adult population, reproductive effects, such as decreased sperm count in men and spontaneous abortions in women have been associated with high lead exposure.
- Acute exposure to lead induces brain damage, kidney damage, and gastrointestinal diseases.
- Chronic exposure may cause adverse effects on the blood, central nervous system, blood pressure, kidneys, and vitamin D metabolism.

- Lead is potentially carcinogenic, inducing renal tumors in rats and mice.
- Prenatal exposure to lead with reduced birth weight and preterm delivery, and with neurodevelopmental abnormalities in offspring.

II) Mercury

Source of exposure
- Dental amalgams - Dental amalgams contain over 50% elemental mercury.
- Fish consumption - Mercury enters water as a natural process of off-gassing from the earth's crust and also through industrial pollution. Algae and bacteria methylate the mercury entering the waterways. Methyl mercury then makes its way through the food chain into fish, shellfish, and eventually into humans.
- Mercury is utilized in the electrical industry (switches, thermostats, batteries), dentistry (dental amalgams), and numerous industrial processes, including the production of caustic soda, in nuclear reactors, as antifungal agents for wood processing, as a solvent for reactive and precious metal, and as a preservative of pharmaceutical products.
- Vaccines include thimerosal, which contains mercury.

Effects of mercury exposure
- All forms of mercury are toxic, and their effects include gastrointestinal toxicity, neurotoxicity, and nephrotoxicity.
- Mercury can induce carcinogenesis
- Mercury is a selenium antagonist and also blocks the intracellular function of zinc - these are the most fundamental elements and catalysts.

The two most highly absorbed species are elemental mercury ($Hg0$) and methyl mercury (MeHg). Dental amalgams contain over 50% elemental mercury. The elemental vapor is highly lipophilic and is effectively absorbed through the lungs and tissues lining the mouth. After

Hg0 enters the blood, it rapidly passes through cell membranes, which include both the blood-brain barrier and the placental barrier. Once it gains entry into the cell, Hg0 is oxidized and becomes highly reactive Hg2+. Methyl mercury derived from eating fish is readily absorbed in the gastrointestinal tract and because of its lipid solubility, can easily cross both the placental and blood-brain barriers. Once mercury is absorbed, it has a very low excretion rate. A major proportion of what is absorbed accumulates in the kidneys, neurological tissue and the liver. All forms of mercury are toxic and their effects include gastrointestinal toxicity, neurotoxicity, and nephrotoxicity.

III) Arsenic

Sources of exposure

- Environmental pollution by arsenic occurs because of natural phenomena such as volcanic eruptions and soil erosion, and anthropogenic activities.
- Several arsenic-containing compounds are produced industrially and have been used to manufacture products with agricultural applications such as insecticides, herbicides, fungicides, algicides, sheep dips, wood preservatives, and dyestuffs.
- Arsenic compounds have also been used in the medical field for at least a century in the treatment of syphilis, yaws, amoebic dysentery, and trypanosomiasis. Arsenic-based drugs are still used in treating certain tropical diseases such as African sleeping sickness and amoebic dysentery, and in veterinary medicine to treat parasitic diseases, including filariasis in dogs and black head in turkeys and chickens.
- Diet, for most individuals, is the largest source of exposure. Its concentration in various foods ranges from 20 to 140 ng/kg.
- Arsenic concentrations in air range from 1 to 3 ng/m3 in remote locations (away from human releases) and from 20 to 100 ng/m3 in cities.
- Arsenic in water concentration is usually less than 10µg/L, although higher levels can occur near natural mineral deposits or mining sites.

Effects of arsenic exposure
- Several epidemiological studies have reported a strong association between arsenic exposure and increased risks of carcinogenesis, especially carcinoma of the bladder, kidney, skin, and liver.
- Systemic effects include cardiovascular and peripheral vascular disease, developmental anomalies, neurologic and neurobehavioral disorders, diabetes, hearing loss, portal fibrosis, hematologic disorders (anemia, leukopenia and eosinophilia) and carcinoma.
- Arsenic exposure affects virtually all organ systems, including the cardiovascular, dermatologic, nervous, hepatobiliary, renal, gastrointestinal, and respiratory systems.
- It can often give rise to neurological irritation symptoms or emotional irritability.

IV) Cadmium

Source of exposure
- Inhalation via cigarette smoke.
- Eating contaminated foods. Foodstuffs rich in cadmium can greatly increase the cadmium concentration in human bodies. Examples are liver, mushrooms, shellfish, mussels, cocoa powder and dried seaweed.
- Inhalation of emissions from industrial activities, including mining, smelting, and manufacturing of batteries, pigments, stabilizers, and alloys.

Effects of Cadmium exposure
- After acute ingestion, symptoms such as abdominal pain, burning sensation, nausea, vomiting, salivation, muscle cramps, vertigo, shock, loss of consciousness and convulsions. Acute cadmium ingestion can also cause gastrointestinal tract erosion, pulmonary, hepatic or renal injury and coma, depending on the route of poisoning.
- Chronic inhalation exposure to cadmium particulates is generally

associated with changes in pulmonary function and chest radiographs consistent with emphysema.
- Workplace exposure to airborne cadmium particulates has been associated with decreases in olfactory function.
- Chronic low-level cadmium exposure is associated with decreases in bone mineral density and osteoporosis.
- Carcinogenesis: there is an association between occupational cadmium exposure and lung cancer. In some studies, occupational or environmental cadmium exposure has also been associated with the development of cancers of the prostate, kidney, liver, hematopoietic system and stomach.

V) Chromium

Source of exposure
- Ingestion of chromium-containing food and water. Most fresh foods typically contain chromium levels ranging from <10 to 1,300 µg/kg.
- Occupational exposure occurs via inhalation. The principal route of human exposure to chromium is through inhalation.

Effects of chromium exposure
- Breathing high levels of chromium can cause irritation to the lining of the nose and nose ulcers.
- Ingestion of chromium can cause irritation and ulcers in the stomach and small intestine.
- Anemia
- Sperm damage and male reproductive system damage.
- Allergic reactions consisting of severe redness and swelling of the skin.
- Acute poisoning from accidental or intentional ingestion of extremely high doses of chromium (VI) compounds by humans has resulted in severe respiratory, cardiovascular, gastrointestinal, hematological, hepatic, renal, and neurological effects as part of the sequelae leading to death.

- An increase in stomach tumors was observed in humans and animals exposed to chromium in drinking water.

Other commonly found toxic heavy metals:
- Tin (Sn) is just as toxic and is contained mostly in amalgam.
- Palladium (Pd) is found in gold fillings (gold filled with alloy).
- Copper found in saliva mainly comes from gold and amalgam fillings that contain it. High copper in the body is caused by chronic inflammation, which can occur in the liver.

CHAPTER 4

Organic Pollutant Exposure in our Environment

Our body's metabolic detoxification is an ongoing process and our organs work to eliminate environmental toxins we come into contact with daily. These can come in the form of toxic bacteria, organic pollutants like plasticizers and heavy metals to name a few. The most common exposure we get is from the foods we ingest daily, especially toxic chemicals from agriculture production like pesticides, herbicides and fertilizers. Besides these chemicals in our foods, we also face these toxins in the environment we come in contact with, for example, the materials used in construction like paint, wood preservation, carpet chemicals, chemical cleaners and shampoos. The plastics we use to wrap and contain our foods are also high in organic pollutants like BPA. To add to that, many of us have dental fillings made of mercury amalgams which, over time, is oxidized by our mouth bacteria and seeps into our body to cause a high mercury burden. Air pollutants are insidiously present in our environment directly from cigarette smoke or from exhaust fumes from cars. Every day, our body faces an onslaught of toxins and chemicals which hitherto from the times of our ancestors were not present before. In times like this, it is even more important to think about optimizing our body's detoxification process to reduce exposure and reduce the risk these toxins can cause to our bodies.

Xenoestrogens - The Endocrine Disruptors
The endocrine system in our body is managed by hormones, and these hormones can affect our growth (the growth hormone), can affect our stress, metabolic rate and energy (the cortisol hormone), and also affect our pubertal growth, our sexual features and pregnancy (the male and

female hormones).

In recent years, endocrine-disrupting hormones (the xenoestrogens) are becoming more and more widespread as these substances are found to disrupt the normal function of our endocrine system. They do this in a few ways:

1. they vie with our own hormones for the receptors and hence reduces the effects of our own hormones.
2. they increase the effects of our hormones by acting like our own hormones and having a stimulating effect on the receptors causing precocious puberty.
3. they act as false messengers and can disrupt the process of reproduction and hence reduce fertility.

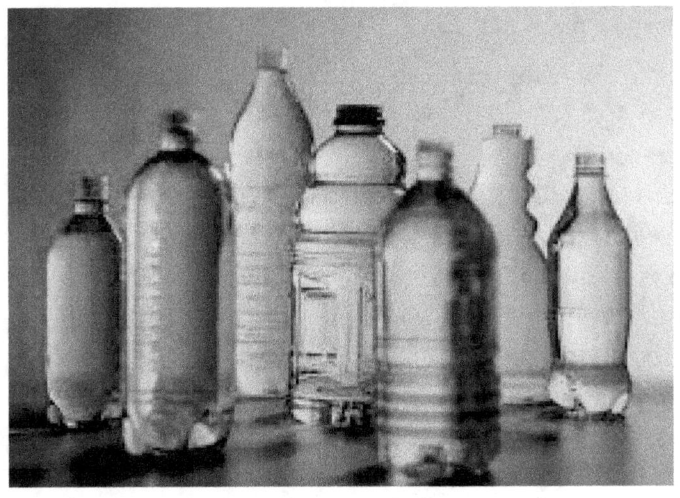

Some of the common estrogen mimickers in our environment include:

Biphenyl (BPA

BPA is being used in the production of plastics and resins. It is also commonly found in canned foods (epoxy resins are used to coat the inside of metal products) and plastic packaging of foods, polycarbonate plastic bottles, cashier's receipts, etc. Some dental sealants and composites also contain BPA.

Steps to reduce your exposure to BPA:
*   Use BPA-free products. In recent years, manufacturers are producing more BPA-free bottles and plastic containers.

- Reduce your intake of canned food products.
- Avoid heating your plastic food containers or food wrapped in plastic films in the microwave oven as this allows BPA to enter our foods.
- Use alternatives like glass bottles instead of plastic.

Phthalates

Phthalates are plasticizer chemicals found in fragrances in shampoos and cleaning agents, plastic toys and plastic wraps. They are also found in personal care products like nail polish, hair sprays, soaps and shampoos, etc. Phthalates exposure has been linked to change in sex hormone levels, altered development of genitals, low sperm count and quality of sperms.

Ways to reduce exposure include:
- avoid plastic food containers, plastic kid's toys and plastic wraps
- avoid using personal products high in fragrances.

Flame Retardants

Flame retardants (PBDEs) are found in mattresses, upholstered furniture, foam cushions, baby car seats, insulation and electronics. These chemicals have been associated with hormone disruption, cancer and even attention deficit disorder in children. The flame retardants can migrate from the products to the indoor air and find their way into our bodies when we inhale or ingest them. Environmental studies have found high levels of flame retardants in Americans nationwide, with children having a greater accumulation than adults.

Ways to reduce your exposure to PBDEs include:
- By-products that are free from flame retardants by checking the packaging
- Wash your hands and fingers regularly, especially for babies who put their fingers into the mouth.
- Vacuum regularly and wipe with a wet cloth regularly to prevent dust that contains flame retardants from accumulating in your home.

Some other chemicals that are xenoestrogens in our environment include:
A) Skincare
- 4-Methylbenzylidene camphor (4-MBC) (sunscreen lotions)

- Parabens
- Benzophenone (sunscreen lotions)

B) Food
- Erythrosine
- Phenosulfothiazine (a red dye)
- BHA (a food preservative)

C) Insecticide
- Atrazine (weed killer)
- DDT (insecticide)
- Dieldrine (insecticide)
- Endosulfan (insecticide)
- Heptachlor (insecticide)
- Lindane (insecticide used to treat liceand scabies)
- Methoxychlor (insecticide)

D) Others
- Chlorine and chlorine by-products
- Alkylphenol (surfactant used in cleaning detergents)

E) Building supplies
- Pentachlorphenol (general biocide and wood preservative)
- Polychlorinated Biphenyls/PCBs (in electrical oils, lubricants, adhesives, paints)

Ways to minimize exposure to xenoestrogens:
1) Food
- Buy organic produce, preferably those grown locally and in-season without preservatives.
- Peel all the non-organic fruits and vegetables.
- Wash the vegetables of all herbicides, pesticides and fungicides.
- Buy hormone-free, antibiotic-free meats and dairy products.

2) Reduce plastic use
- Do not microwave food in plastic containers or use plastic wraps in the microwave.
- Use glass or ceramics to store foods.

- Do not leave plastic containers, especially bottled drinking water in the sun.
- Don't refill plastic water bottles.

3) Household products
- Use chemical-free, biodegradable household cleaning products where possible.
- Choose chlorine-free and unbleached paper products (tampons, menstrual pads, toilet paper, etc.)
- Use a chlorine filter on showerheads and filter your drinking water.

4) Health and beauty products
- Avoid creams and cosmetics that contain parabens.
- Minimize exposure to nail polish and nail polish removers.
- Use naturally based fragrances like essential oils.
- Use chemical-free natural soaps and shampoos.

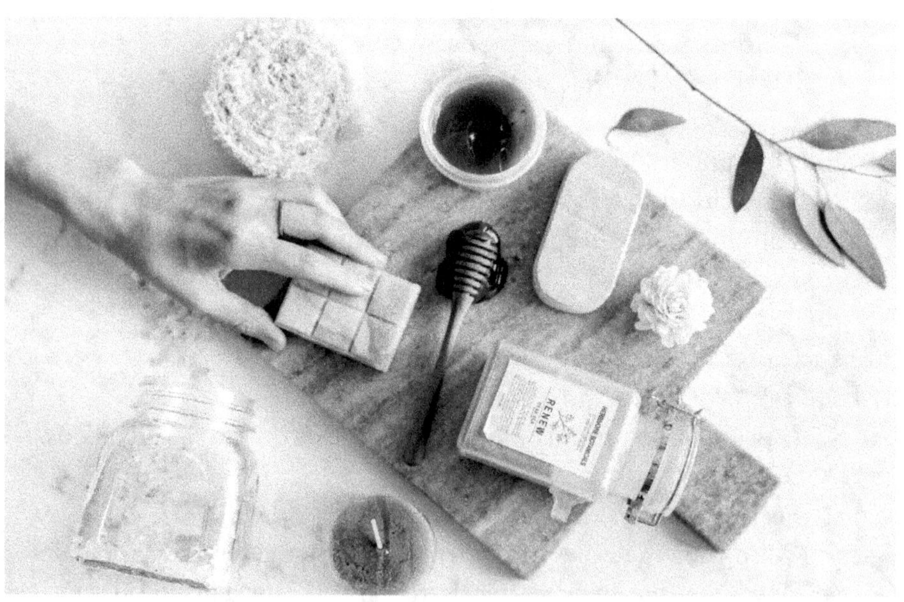

5) At the workplace
- Be aware and avoid exposure to flame retardant products.
- Avoid noxious gas from copiers and printers, carpets, etc.

CHAPTER 5

Dental interference field and toxicity

Interference fields and neural therapy

Besides interfering with the cell membrane potential, which could affect the nervous system, heavy metals could also create interference fields. Interference fields are studied in biological medicine and came from a modality developed in Germany called neural therapy. These are electrical fields generated by old scars, injuries, and residua of dental procedures that leave certain bodily energies "blocked" and unable to heal, hence creating energetic disturbances. Understanding the interference fields allows us to apply methods to release these blockages and allow the body to reboot and for the meridians to flow more readily. It is hypothesised this phenomenon is regulated by the autonomic nervous system and hence injecting procaine into these interference fields to unblock the system is called neural therapy.

Researchers discovered that interference fields were created due to a disruption in the normal resting cell membrane potential. In normal healthy cells, there is a -70mV difference inside the cell relative to the outside of the cell. As the cells become abnormal, the resting cell membrane potential deviates from -70mV. This change in potential causes less oxygen and nutrients to enter the cell and also more waste products to accumulate within the cell.

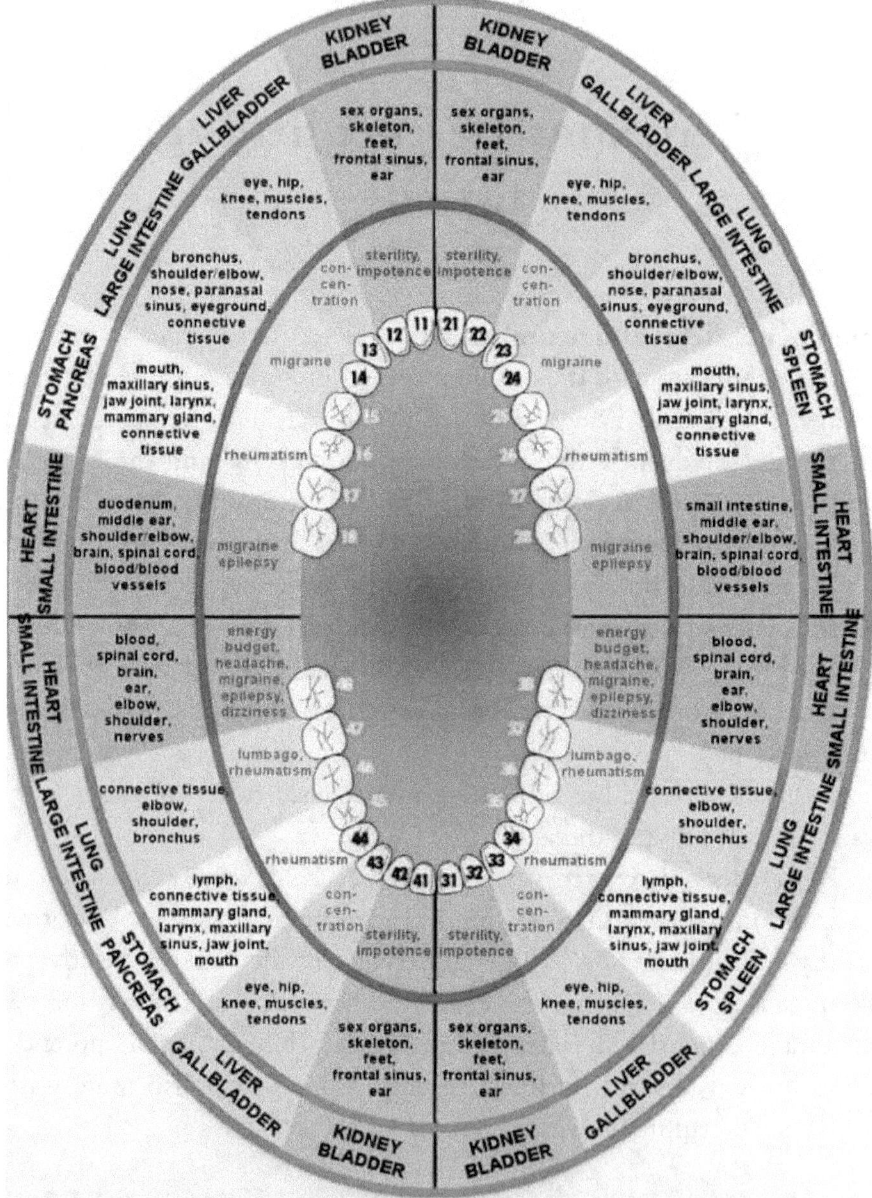

KIDNEY BLADDER
KIDNEY BLADDER
LIVER GALLBLADDER
LIVER GALLBLADDER LARGE INTESTINE
LARGE INTESTINE GALLBLADDER
LUNG
LUNG
STOMACH PANCREAS
STOMACH SPLEEN
HEART SMALL INTESTINE
HEART SMALL INTESTINE
HEART SMALL INTESTINE
HEART SMALL INTESTINE
LUNG LARGE INTESTINE
LUNG LARGE INTESTINE
STOMACH PANCREAS
STOMACH SPLEEN
LIVER GALLBLADDER
LIVER GALLBLADDER
KIDNEY BLADDER
KIDNEY BLADDER
sex organs, skeleton, feet, frontal sinus, ear
sex organs, skeleton, feet, frontal sinus, ear
eye, hip, knee, muscles, tendons
eye, hip, knee, muscles, tendons
sterility, impotence
sterility, impotence
concentration
concentration
bronchus, shoulder/elbow, nose, paranasal sinus, eyeground, connective tissue
bronchus, shoulder/elbow, nose, paranasal sinus, eyeground, connective tissue
migraine
migraine
mouth, maxillary sinus, jaw joint, larynx, mammary gland, connective tissue
mouth, maxillary sinus, jaw joint, larynx, mammary gland, connective tissue
rheumatism
rheumatism
duodenum, middle ear, shoulder/elbow, brain, spinal cord, blood/blood vessels
small intestine, middle ear, shoulder/elbow, brain, spinal cord, blood/blood vessels
migraine epilepsy
migraine epilepsy
blood, spinal cord, brain, ear, elbow, shoulder, nerves
blood, spinal cord, brain, ear, elbow, shoulder, nerves
energy budget, headache, migraine, epilepsy, dizziness
energy budget, headache, migraine, epilepsy, dizziness
lumbago, rheumatism
lumbago, rheumatism
connective tissue, elbow, shoulder, bronchus
connective tissue, elbow, shoulder, bronchus
rheumatism
rheumatism
lymph, connective tissue, mammary gland, larynx, maxillary sinus, jaw joint, mouth
lymph, connective tissue, mammary gland, larynx, maxillary sinus, jaw joint, mouth
concentration
concentration
sterility, impotence
sterility, impotence
eye, hip, knee, muscles, tendons
eye, hip, knee, muscles, tendons
sex organs, skeleton, feet, frontal sinus, ear
sex organs, skeleton, feet, frontal sinus, ear
11 21
12 22
13 23
14 24
15 25
16 26
17 27
18 28
44 34
43 33
42 32
41 31

Meridian Tooth Chart

	1	2	3	4	5	6	7	8	9	10	11	12	13	14	15	16
Joints	Right: Shoulder, elbow, hand (ulnar), S.I. joint, foot, toes	Right: TMJ, anterior hip/knee, medial ankle		Right: Shoulder-elbow-hand (radial), foot, big toe		Right: Posterior knee, hip, lateral ankle	Right: Posterior knee, sacro, coccygeal joint, posterior ankle		Left: Posterior knee, sacro, coccygeal joint, posterior ankle		Left: Posterior knee, hip, lateral ankle	Left: Shoulder-elbow-hand (radial), foot, big toe		Left: TMJ, anterior hip/knee, medial ankle		Left: Shoulder-elbow-hand (ulnar), S.I. joint, foot, toes
Mammary Glands		R i g h t B r e a s t										L e f t B r e a s t				
Endocrine Glands	Anterior pituitary	Parathyroid	Thyroid	Thymus	Posterior pituitary	Intermediate lobe of pituitary	Pineal		Pineal		Intermediate lobe of pituitary	Posterior pituitary	Thymus	Thyroid	Parathyroid	Anterior pituitary
Organs	Right heart, right duodenum, ileum, terminal ileum	Pancreas, right side of stomach, esophagus		Right lung, right side of large intestine		Right side of liver, gall bladder, right side of biliary ducts	Right kidney, bladder, ureters, prostate, rectum, anus		Left kidney, bladder, ureters, prostate, rectum, anus		Left side of liver, biliary ducts	Left lung, left side of large intestine		Spleen, left side of stomach, esophagus		Left heart, left side of duodenum, jejunum, ileum
Teeth Pictured (Retromolar)																(Retromolar)
Names of Teeth	Right upper 3rd molar (wisdom)	Right upper 2nd molar	Right upper 1st molar	Right upper 2nd bicuspid (pre-molar)	Right upper 1st bicuspid (pre-molar)	Right upper canine (cuspid)	Right upper lateral incisor	Right upper central incisor	Left upper central incisor	Left upper lateral incisor	Left upper canine (cuspid)	Left upper 1st bicuspid (pre-molar)	Left upper 2nd bicuspid (pre-molar)	Left upper 1st molar	Left upper 2nd molar	Left upper 3rd molar (wisdom)
American Nomenclature	1	2	3	4	5	6	7	8	9	10	11	12	13	14	15	16
	32	31	30	29	28	27	26	25	24	23	22	21	20	19	18	17
Names of Teeth	Right lower 3rd molar (wisdom)	Right lower 2nd molar	Right lower 1st molar	Right lower 2nd bicuspid (pre-molar)	Right lower 1st bicuspid (pre-molar)	Right lower canine (cuspid)	Right lower lateral incisor	Right lower central incisor	Left lower central incisor	Left lower lateral incisor	Left lower canine (cuspid)	Left lower 1st bicuspid (pre-molar)	Left lower 2nd bicuspid (pre-molar)	Left lower 1st molar	Left lower 2nd molar	Left lower 3rd molar (wisdom)
Teeth Pictured (Retromolar)																(Retromolar)
Organs	Right heart, terminal ileum, ileo-cecal	Pancreas, right side of stomach, pylorus, esophagus		Right lung, right side of large intestine		Right side of liver, gall bladder, right side of biliary ducts	Right kidney, bladder, uterus, prostate, rectum, anus		Left kidney, bladder, uterus, prostate, rectum, anus		Left side of liver, biliary ducts	Left lung, left side of large intestine		Spleen, left side of stomach, esophagus		Left heart, left side of pancreas, ileum
Endocrine Glands				Ovaries		testicles	Adrenals		Adrenals		Ovaries	testicles				
Mammary glands		R i g h t B r e a s t										L e f t B r e a s t				
Joints	Right: Shoulder, elbow, hand (ulnar), S.I. joint, foot, toes	Right: TMJ, anterior hip/knee, medial ankle		Right: Shoulder-elbow-hand (radial), foot, big toe		Right: Posterior knee, hip, lateral ankle	Right: Posterior knee, sacro, coccygeal joint, posterior ankle		Left: Posterior knee, sacro, coccygeal joint, posterior ankle		Left: Posterior knee, hip, lateral ankle	Left: Shoulder-elbow-hand (radial), foot, big toe		Left: TMJ, anterior hip/knee, medial ankle		Left: Shoulder-elbow-hand (ulnar), S.I. joint, foot, toes

http://biocompatibledentist.org/holistic_dentistry/tooth-chart/

The most common interference fields are caused mainly by scars, ganglia and organs. Scars can arise from surgical procedures, or from cuts, piercings and tattoos. Scars create a problem when they develop abnormal resting cell membrane potential that becomes interference fields. In Traditional Chinese Medicine, this is similar to blocking the flow of the Qi or energy through the meridians.

In the chronic sick, it is common to find interference fields originating in the teeth. It is believed that each tooth sits on an acupuncture meridian. For example, the wisdom teeth connect to the heart and small intestine meridians. Interference fields that develop after removal of wisdom teeth or when a root canal is placed on the wisdom tooth area can lead to heart and digestive disorders. These are the main causes of dental interference fields: mercury amalgams, cavitation, and root canals. Mercury amalgams, especially those that have been placed in the mouth for many years and have been oxidised, is a known toxic heavy metal that could create a whole host of health issues. These fillings appear as gray or silver irregular amalgams in the mouth. There has been lots of literature written about the harmful effects of mercury amalgams yet sadly, few people are aware that their symptoms could have originated from their amalgams in the mouth. If the mercury amalgam is a likely source of the dental interference field, it would have to be removed preferably by a trained biological dentist to ensure the safe removal of the mercury. The very sick patients should not undergo amalgam removal unless under the care of a highly qualified biological dentist as some mercury can leak out during the procedure and can trigger high levels of inflammation. Also, these patients need to be closely monitored before and after the amalgam removal. The key to safe removal and optimal results are prepared timing, adequate preparation, and close monitoring after the removal to ensure the metals don't cause more inflammation in the body.

The other dental issues that can disrupt the interference fields are cavitation and root canals. Cavitation may create areas of dead bone in the jaw if there is poor healing, also known as osteonecrosis. This differs from cavities where there is simply a breakdown of the enamel. These areas of dead bone can create pockets of chronic bacterial infections causing interference fields and also inflammation to occur in the body. Wisdom tooth extraction sites and even root canal sites are frequent sites where cavitation can develop.

Trained biological dentists treat cavitation by injecting medical ozone into the gums over the cavitation. The other option is to use the traditional surgical curettage to drain any infections or abscesses in the jawbone.

Root canals are another source of dental interference field. Root canals inserted can never be completely sterile and thus pockets of bacteria will remain around the root canaled tooth creating an interference field. The only definitive treatment is to remove the root canal tooth and use Ozone to treat the infected gums and jawbone.

Somatotopical connections of the teeth

Teeth	Meridien association	Organs
All front teeth	Kidney bladder meridien	Ears, sacrum, sacroiliac joint, kidneys, bladder, vertebrae L2, genitalia
All canine teeth	Gallbladder – liver meridien	Bile, liver, eyes, maxillary joints
Upper molars, upper and lower pre-molars	Stomach-spleen-pancreas meridien	Stomach, pancreas, front of knee, thyroid, breast
Upper premolars	Large intestine – lung merdien	Colon, lungs, part of maxillary sinus, cervical spine, shoulder
All wisdom teeth	Small intestine – heart meridien	Mastoid process, small intestine, vertebrae T4, heart, back of shoulder, head, lips.

Factors that cause mercury to be released from amalgam fillings

1) Acidic pH of the saliva

- the more acidic the saliva, the greater the release of mercury. Hence, taking an alkalizing diet or alkaline supplements would help to prevent the leakage from the amalgams.

2) Age and surface structure of the filling

- The rougher the surface of the amalgam, the greater the area, and hence more mercury is released when it comes into contact with our saliva and foods.

3) Galvanic activity in the mouth

- Mixtures of metals in the mouth create free electrons causing galvanic currents to be created in the mouth. This is especially worse with root canal fillings or root pins below the amalgam fillings.

4) Nicotine and acidic food

- When a person smokes cigarette, it causes about 100 times more mercury to be released. Nicotine acid is a powerful mercury solvent and can cause this leakage of mercury.

5) Mechanical overload

- chewing gums create a mechanical pulling force that pulls mercury more easily out from the amalgams.

Proper removal of amalgams to prevent heavy metal toxicity

Removal of amalgam preferably must be done by a properly trained biological dentist. If amalgams are removed the wrong way, it will cause high levels of heavy metal intoxication in the body.

Important measures to note includes:
- Every removal of amalgams must be accompanied by an elimination program (see Amalgam Elimination Program below).
- Removal of amalgam should be done by a properly trained biological dentist using protective measures, including a slow drill and special sanction disposal with a cleaning up system.
- The eliminative treatment using natural supplements may take weeks or months.

The Amalgam Elimination Program

1) Preparation before amalgam removal

Supplements to take:
- Vitamin C 500mg - 3000mg daily
- Zinc tablets 15mg once a day for a month, then take a 1-2 weeks

break. Muscle weakness and tiredness may be a sign of overdose.
- Selenium 150mcg daily
- additional supplements for detox, including chlorella or spirulina.

2) Timing the removal of the amalgam

Removal of the amalgam should be carried out after the patient has been started on the above antioxidant supplements. The removal should be carried out by a slow drill as too high speeds can result in a high temperature and the generation of mercury vapor.

3) Supplements given during the time of removal
- Keep the same supplements as above.
- Dosage of vitamin C should be doubled for a week starting the day before the removal.
- Before and during the amalgam removal, patients are encouraged to alkalinize their bodies by eating more vegetables, avoiding sugars, chewing gums, smoking and eating acidic fruits. The amount of mercury dissolved out of the amalgam fillings depends directly on the acidity of the saliva.

4) After the amalgam removal
- The Elimination Program continues a few months after the removal. It can take up to 4-18months for the more severe cases.
- Continue the basic supplements:
- Vitamin C 500-3000mg /day
- Selenium 150mcg per day
- Zinc 15mg daily for a month, then break for 2 weeks.
- DMSA tabs 100mg one a week up to 6-8 weeks. This is given in cases with strong symptoms and high readings. Make sure patient maintains proper hydration and takes a good mineral supplement as minerals are also removed by DMSA.

Optional:

- Chlorella is a form of algae that helps bind heavy metals and excrete them in the stools. Take 4-5 tabs 3 times a day with plenty of water before meals.
- Spirulina
- Amino acids such as Methionine 1-2g /day
- N-acetyl-cysteine (NAC) 400-600mg two times a day

CHAPTER 6

Methods of detoxification – daily home detoxification

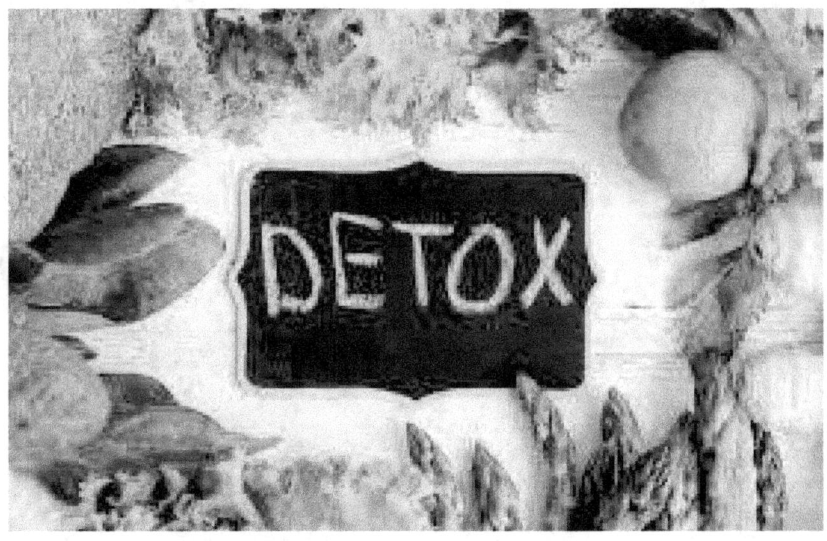

Detoxification can start even at home and it is good to cultivate a habit of doing regular detoxification as our bodies are always exposed to heavy metals in our environment. Daily detoxification helps your body to reduce the accumulation of these toxins in your body and not overwhelm the detoxification process in the liver. This is especially important for people with unhealthy lifestyle habits like drinking alcohol and smoking, where you are introducing more toxins to the liver.

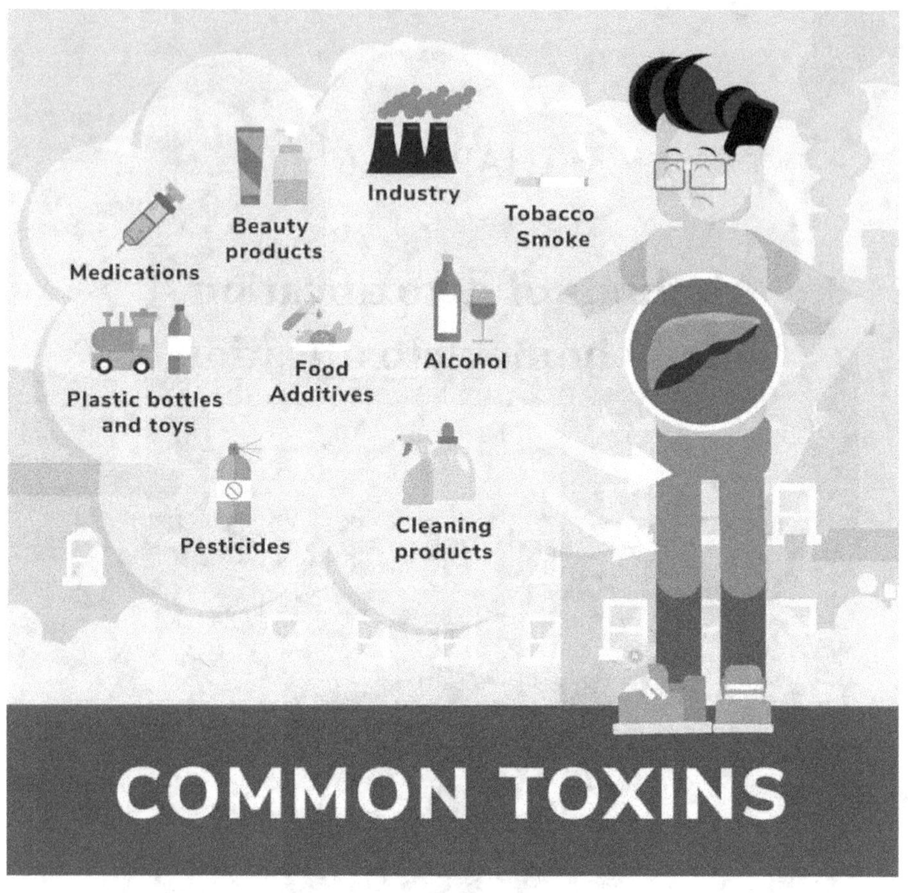

COMMON TOXINS

Methods of detoxification you can do include:

- Find the source and remove or minimize exposure to the heavy metals.
- Remove sources of organic pollutants at home like chemical cleaning agents and shampoos and switch to natural cleaning agents and shampoos.
- Increase your intake of detoxifying foods like cruciferous vegetables, onions, garlic, green tea, cilantro.
- Increase your intake of antioxidants by eating more phytonutrients like colorful vegetables, fruits with high vitamin C.
- Fiber is good for pulling heavy metals out from your stools. Increase your fiber intake through foods like flax or chia seeds, eating more vegetables and legumes, eat more brown alternatives

like brown rice, quinoa. Or simply buying Psyllium Husk from your supplement store to add into your smoothie or oats. Also, make sure that you have good bowel output to excrete the heavy metals.

- Go for infra-red saunas two to three times a week, each session about 15 minutes to sweat out the heavy metals. Then immediately after that, take a cold shower to wash off the heavy metals in your sweat.

- Try to increase alkalinity of the body, which helps detoxification by switching to a more vegetarian and plant-based diet. Also, taking warm water with a piece of lemon in the morning is a good way of alkaline in your body.

- Amino acids are needed to boost phase 2 detoxification in the liver. Consume clean organic meats like grass-fed beef, lamb, lean pork and organic hormone-free chicken. If eating processed meats like bacon, sausages, get them from local farmers, usually without much preservatives or additives. Quality proteins can also be obtained from plant proteins like beans and legumes, nuts and seeds.

- Optimize your intake of minerals such as selenium from Brazil nuts, B vitamins from various food sources or supplements to encourage phase I liver detoxification.

- Take binders like psyllium husk, charcoal, Zeolite or cholestyramine to help mind heavy metals out from the stools.

- For detoxification, drink lots of water daily or detox teas or green teas, which also contain high antioxidant levels.

- Adding natural products like Chlorella or Spirulina into your juice or supplements can also naturally help to bind heavy metals out of the body.

- Avoid high mercury fishes like big sea tuna, farmed salmon, grouper, King Mackerel and swordfish. See the FDA fish consumer guide www.fda.gov/food/consumers/advice-about-eating-fish

- If you drink, try to buy organic sources of coffee beans and alcohol as these drinks usually contain toxins from the environment and can accumulate daily in our body if we drink them regularly.

Nutrients Used for Detox

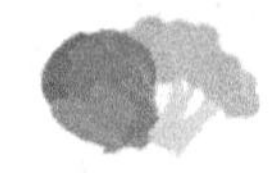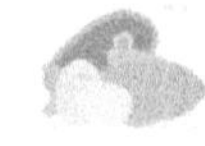

B vitamins
Vitmamin C
Glutathione
Choline
Silymarin (Milk Thistle)
Flavonoids
Glucosinolates
Curcumin
N-Acetyl-Cysteine
Glycine
Iron, Selenium, Zinc, Copper, Magnesium

...and many more
(depending on your gene variants)

Whole Foods that Support Detox

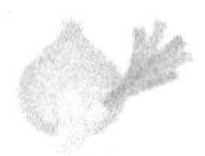

Cruciferous
vegetables
and their sprouts

Grass-fed meat,
eggs and
low-mercury fish

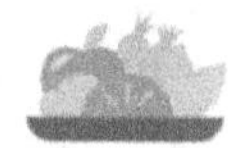

Allium
Vegetables

Low-glycemic
berries, fruits and
vegetables

If you have mercury amalgams, they are usually the source of high mercury in the body and with oxidation happening daily in our mouth, this mercury can slowly seep into our body and cause toxic effects on the nervous system, the brain or the rest of the body. Find a biological dentist who can safely help to remove the mercury amalgam as unsafe removal can sometimes release mercury into the body and cause a potential health risk when absorbed into the body.

Other lifestyles tips for reducing our toxic exposure:
- avoid plastic wraps/containers
- avoid microwaving your foods
- avoid deep frying your foods, try steaming, boiling, baking and. shallow frying
- minimize exposure to EMF radiation. Put your phones on airplane mode when you sleep at night and limit phone usage to minimum hours per day. If you have to use your phones and computers for long hours daily due to work, wear glasses that help to screen off the blue light.

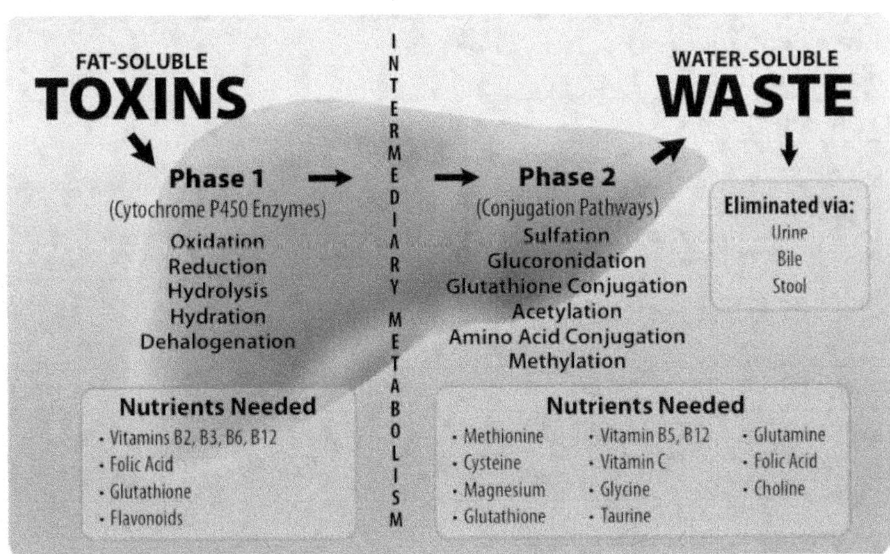

Supplements to boost detoxification

Pre-treatment	
ToxEase GL (from Body Balance)	1 drop 2 times daily
Gallbladder – improving the ability to make bile	
Acetyl-L-carnitine	500mg 2 times daily
Phosphatidylcholine	400mg up to 1200mg per day
Oxbile	125mg to 500mg 1-2 time per day
Calcium pyruvate	750mg 1-2 times per day
Gallbladder – improving the ability to mobilize bile	
Bitters	2 pumps 1-3 times per day
Artichoke	400mg 1-3 times per day
Milk Thistle	250mg 1-3 times daily
Coffee enemas	

Liver - enhancing detoxification	
Milk Thistle	250mg 1-3 times per day
Alpha Lipoic Acid	100 – 200mg 2 times a day
NAC	500mg 2 times a day
Artichoke extract	500mg 2 times per day
Indole-3-carbinol	200mg 2 times daily
Gut	
Probiotics to repopulate gut	
Fiber	

Medical Detoxification

Chelation comes from the Greek word "Chee" which means claw.

Chelation therapy is a process whereby the chemical compound EDTA or DMPS is injected intravenously into the bloodstream to draw out the heavy metals from the body. But in the process, other minerals may also be drawn out of the body too. When these substances are injected into the body, they grab hold of the metals and minerals such as lead, mercury, copper, iron, arsenic, aluminum and calcium and excrete them out of the money through the bowels or the kidneys.

EDTA (ethylenediaminmnetetraacetic acid)

EDTA is an FDA-approved method to treat lead poisoning. Some physicians have used IV EDTA to treat coronary artery disease and atherosclerosis, although this form of treatment is still controversial. Proponents of this method believe that EDTA, which usually binds with the calcium in the bones, also acts to bind calcium deposits from plaques in the arteries and this helps to "clean out" the calcium plaques from the arteries and reduce risk of heart disease.

There is a recent study to show the effectiveness of EDTA therapy for preventing cardiovascular events, especially in diabetic patients with a history of heart attack. In 2002, the National Institute of Health did a big study on chelation therapy called TACT. The Trial to Assess Chelation Therapy (TACT), found a 40% reduction in total mortality, 40% reduction in recurrent heart attacks and about 50% reduction in overall mortality in patients with diabetes who previously suffered from a heart attack. But it only worked in people with diabetes. The study didn't find enough proof that it treats heart disease and hence hitherto, the FDA has not approved this treatment for treating heart disease. TACT was a large, randomized, placebo-controlled study published in JAMA that randomized patients to a series of IV chelation using EDTA or placebo. (16)

Some patients report reduced pain from chronic inflammatory diseases like arthritis, as it acts as an antioxidant to remove inflammatory processes in the body.

Some of the negative side effects of EDTA therapy include kidney damage at high doses, or high blood pressure, headache, and rashes. Monitor the renal function during the IV EDTA chelation treatment. Some patients who have had chelation therapy also have low calcium levels in the blood and it not monitored properly may lead to kidney damage.

In addition, EDTA, besides pulling out heavy metals from the body, also removes vital minerals from the body, including calcium. Supplement the patient with vitamins and minerals to keep them from losing these minerals in the process of chelation.

DMPS

Another intravenous agent used for mercury detoxification is called DMPS (2,3-Dimercapto-1-propanesulfonic acid). It belongs to the thiol group, which binds metals to sulfhydryl groups. It has been registered in Germany since 1997 and is available as a prescription item in various countries. DMPS is routinely used as an antidote for heavy metal poisoning and to treat chronic metal overexposure. DMPS is listed as an antidote for treating arsenic, lead and mercury intoxication. DMPS provocation tests are used by physicians before initiating treatment to diagnose the severity of the heavy metal burden in the body.

While chelating agents are officially used for the diagnosis and treatment of an acute heavy metal intoxication, the use of chelating agents for the diagnosis and treatment of a chronic heavy metal burden is not yet fully accepted in the conventional medical field.

Chelating agents have a strong affinity for metals, including the nutrient metals. For DMPS, it has a strong copper-binding ability, EDTA binds strongly to zinc and calcium. If the patient's nutritional status is not evaluated, the prolonged use of chelating agents can lead to certain mineral deficiencies. Hence during chelation treatment, physicians should closely monitor the patient's nutritional status and supplement or replace deficient nutrients as necessary before starting or during the chelation treatment.

In certain patients who are symptomatic but with unbelievably low levels of heavy metals after the challenge, it may be worthwhile to stimulate bile drainage with Solidago, Vitamin C, Selenium and Zinc for about a month and repeat the test, which often you would find a higher value. This is likely that the patient is a bile excretor and eliminates mercury predominantly via the stools and giving sulphurous, bile-accessible substances such as wild garlic or coriander would loosen the heavy metal from its deep fixation and mobilize it better for elimination.

Genetic ability to detoxify

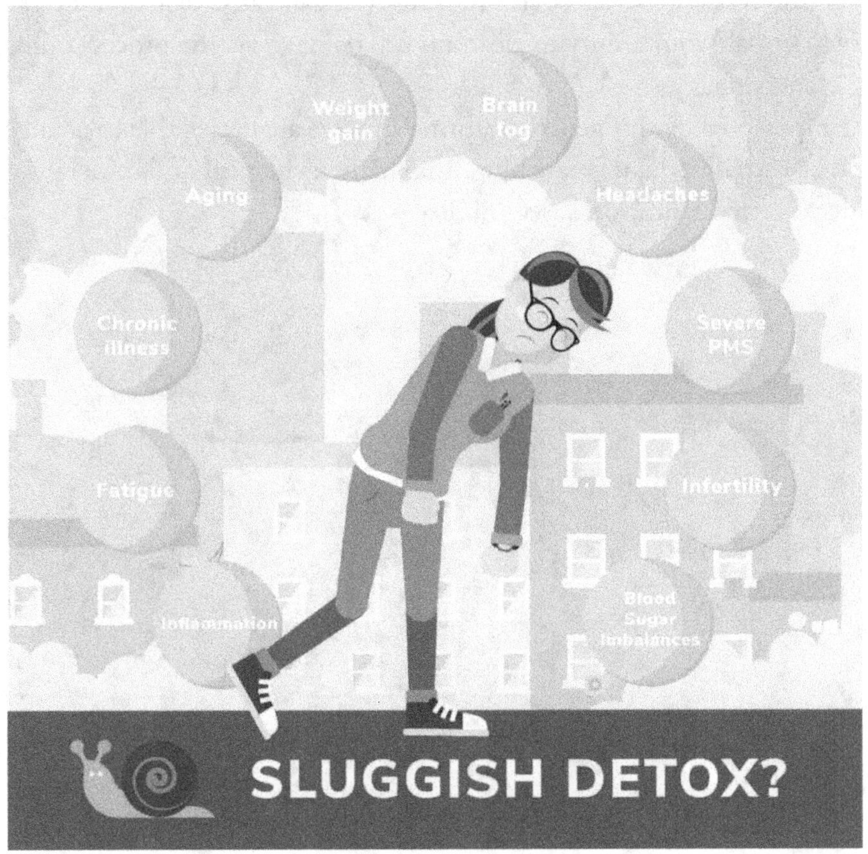

Why do some people not experience any symptoms, but some experience a severe headache, nausea or sickness after exposure to chemicals, cigarette smoke or perfume? The answer lies in your genetic predisposition for detoxification. Some of the common detoxification SNPs to look out for include: MTHFR A1298, ME1, HFE, SLC40A1, CP, SOD1, SOD2, SOD3, CAT, GSR, ULK1, ULK2, ATG 13. Genetics determine how many free radicals you create or whether you are genetically predisposed to oxidative stress. Genetics also determine a cell cleansing process called autophagy, which determines how well a person clears out toxins from the body. We look for detoxification genes that could:

- Affect a person's ability to produce antioxidants to protect you from free radicals and toxins. Superoxide dismutase (SOD), catalase, glutathione, and Nrf2 are SNPs that control the production of good antioxidants.
- Increase the levels of free radicals that can cause oxidative stress.
- Impair your ability to clean up cell damage via the process called autophagy.

Empowered by this genetic information, we are better able to change our diet and lifestyle, increase our antioxidants, vitamins and minerals to reduce our detoxification susceptibility.

Gut Symptoms and Toxicity

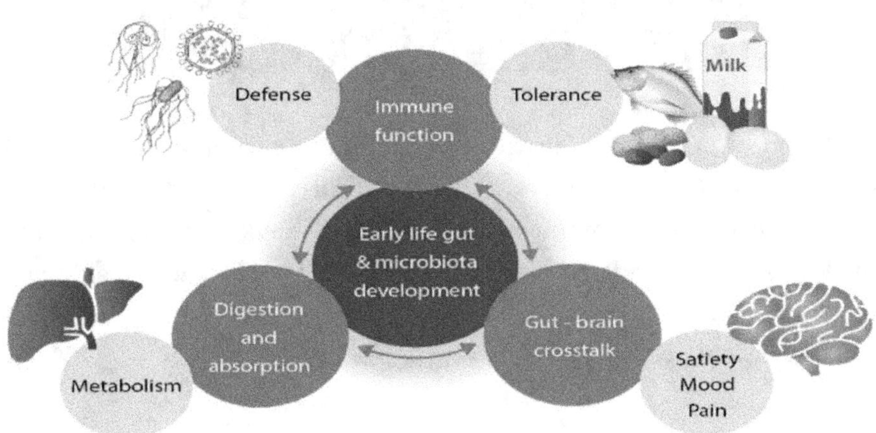

The small intestine excretes about 20L of intestinal mucus a day, which aids in detoxification. Most of the fluid is reabsorbed in the large intestine. Intestinal bacteria/flora helps to retain these excretory substances in the lumen of the intestine, preventing reabsorption or re-intoxication back into the intestinal wall. They bind the toxins and heavy metals and excrete them via the stools.

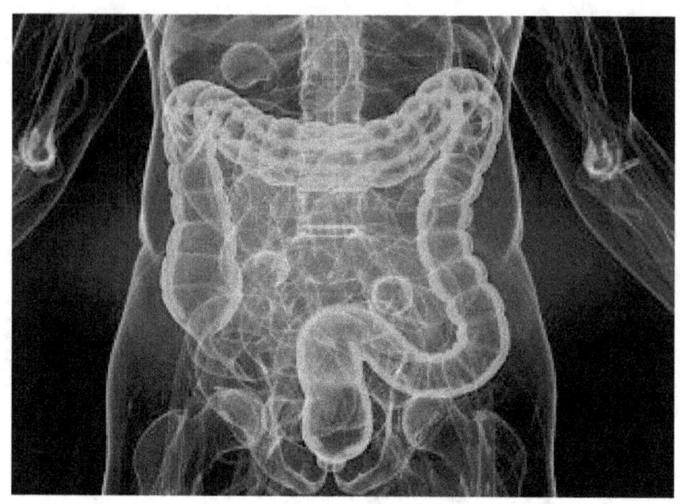

The intestinal mucosa also forms hormone or enzyme-like substances, which controls the motility of the gut and controls the autonomic nervous system (via substances like serotonin, amylase, histamine, etc.). The vagus nerve (the parasympathetic nervous system) is found along the intestinal tract and controls vital functions such as breathing, heartbeat, sleep, intestinal peristalsis, etc.

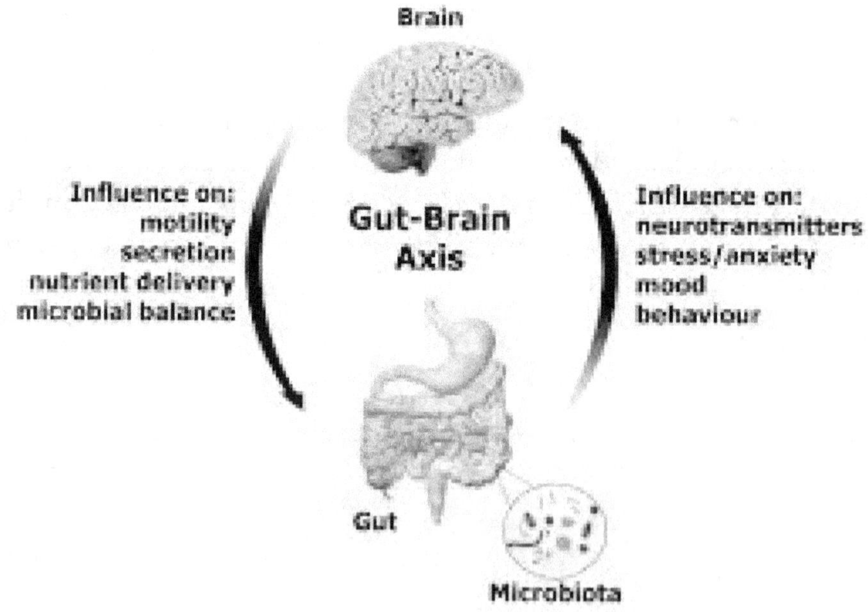

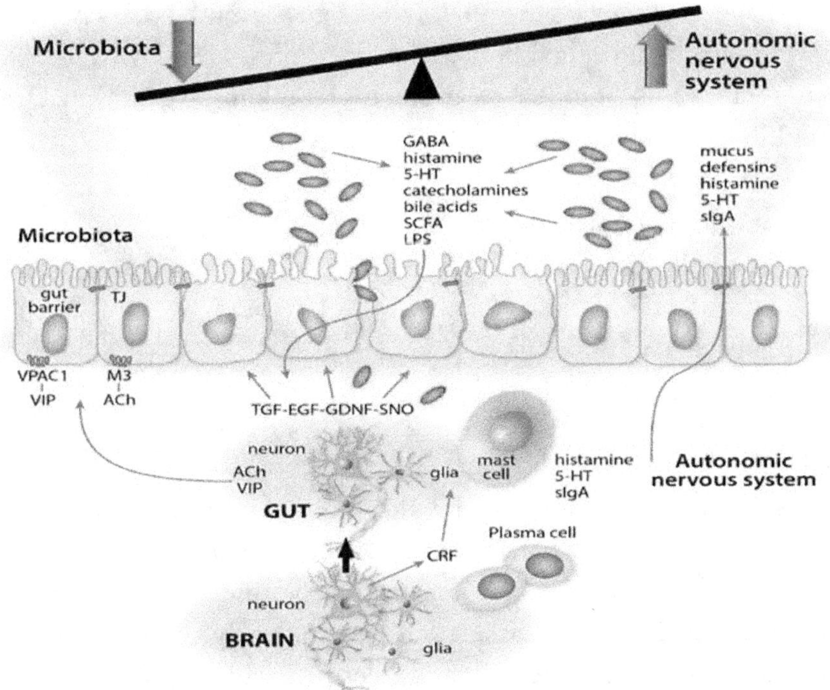

The intestinal tract also controls a major part of our immune system via Peyer's patches, which are tiny lymphoid follicles lining the gut mucosa and it forms almost 80% of our lymphocytic immune system.

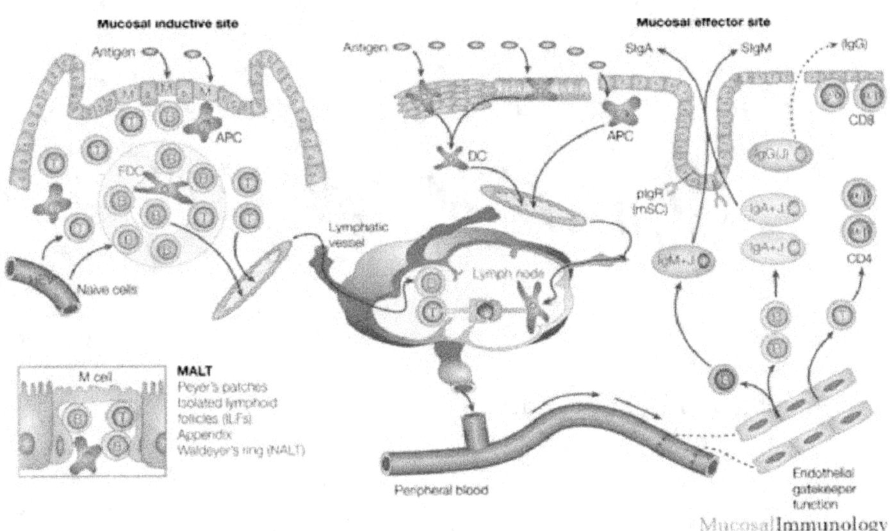

This points to the fact that maintaining good health is closely related to having healthy intestinal flora and proper intestinal activity. The first step is usually to do intestinal cleansing for rebuilding the intestinal tract and building up the immunity.

The main causes of a sick gut include:
- Food allergies
- Gut bacteria, virus, yeast or parasites dysbiosis
- Poor diet and lifestyle
- Heavy metal toxicity

LEAKY GUT

Many substances are taken up by the mucosal cells and transported from there into the mesenchymal cells of the intestinal wall. When the intestinal wall is unhealthy and "leaky", trace elements are less likely to be absorbed, while toxic substances can seep through more easily. The patient absorbs toxic molecules and allergens which puts him/her in immunological overload.

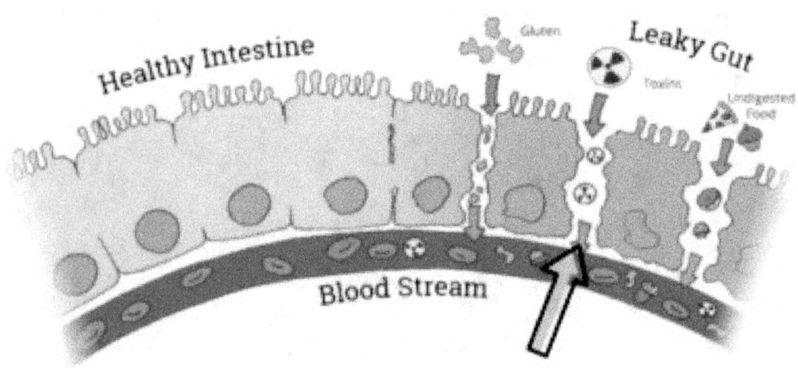

Symptoms of leaky gut include:
- Chronic and recurring allergies
- Fatigue
- Unexplained body aches and headaches
- Poor immune system with tendency to have recurrent infections
- Present with multiple food allergies on the IgG4 screening test.

Causes of leaky gut include:
- Heavy metal toxicity, especially cadmium and mercury
- A diet too low in carbohydrates (too few long-chain carbs from vegetables)
- Trace element deficiency: molybdenum, manganese
- Amino acid deficiency: glutamine, leucine, isoleucine
- Vitamin A and vitamin K deficiency
- Gut infections e.g. Clostridia and Klebsiella can damage the intestinal wall mucosa and protective glycocalyx
- Chemical pollutants from detergents and cleaning agents find their way into our foods and can also destroy the intestinal lining

The investigation for leaky gut involves doing a comprehensive stool analysis to look for gut infections that are present, and also an investigation for digestive enzyme deficiencies, inflammation or raised zonulin as a marker for gut leakiness.

Treatment for leaky gut
- Remove source of heavy metal contamination (i.e., amalgam removal)
- Treat any underlying gut infections with natural antimicrobials
- Take a good multimineral supplement
- Glutamine 2-3 times a day for gut wall repair
- Molybdenum 2mg per day and zinc 30mg per day
- Rebuilding the intestinal bacteria with a good probiotic will help to bind toxins and excrete them in the stool. Having a good diet builds up the intestinal flora - this includes a diet high in minerals, vegetable fibre, and nutritious oils providing good quality fatty acids.

GUT AND TOXICITY

I) History of exposure

A history of exposure is the most critical aspect of diagnosing gut symptoms related to heavy metal toxicity. A complete history includes questions about potential occupational exposures, hobbies, recreational activities, and potential environmental exposure.

A complete dietary history should be taken, especially the ingestion of fish, seafood, and seaweed products since these will frequently be implicated as dietary sources of organic (and relatively nontoxic) mercury, arsenic, or both. The timing of ingestion relative to the collection of urine samples is critical to interpreting the results.

Herbal medications and dietary supplements are also potential sources of heavy metal exposure. Many Ayurvedic and Chinese patent medicines contain heavy metals.

Most acute presentations of heavy metal toxicity involve industrial exposure.

The ingestion of nonfood items such as paint chips, toys, and ballistic devices has also been implicated as the source of metal exposure in several cases.

Retained lead shot may ultimately lead to toxicity as well, although generally, the shot must be bathed in relatively acidic body compartments such as the peritoneal fluid, pleural fluid, cerebrospinal fluid, or synovial fluid for significant absorption of metal ions to occur.

II) Presentation

Lead (Pb) and Cadmium (Cd) are two widespread, non-essential, heavy-metal pollutants of environmental health concern in both industrialized and developing countries. Humans can be exposed to Cd and/or Pb from a variety of sources resulting from past and ongoing anthropogenic activities (industrial emissions, car exhaust fumes, fossil fuel combustion, metallurgy and sea pollution). In particular, smoking and dietary intake (through contaminated cereals, fish, shellfish and drinking water) are the major sources of Cd/Pb entry into the gastrointestinal tract. It is also noteworthy that a large proportion of inhaled Cd ends up in the gastrointestinal tract as a result of mucociliary clearance. Heavy metal exposure is harmful because of acute poisoning on the one hand and long-term toxicity (due to accumulation) on the other.

III) Treatment of gut symptoms related to toxicity

If the gut symptoms are present due to high levels of toxins in the body, it is of primary importance to detoxify the patient of heavy metals. Environmental toxins like heavy metals and organic pollutants and mycotoxins from molds can damage the mucosal lining of the intestines and increase intestinal permeability leading to "leaky gut". As the gut becomes more permeable, the intestinal tract becomes inflamed and allows larger undigested food particles or toxins or bacterial or viral endotoxins to pass through, leading to a weakened immune system, which becomes overstimulated. This can lead to allergies, autoimmune conditions or even inflammatory joint conditions like arthritis. The toxins that pass through the gut wall go to the liver, which becomes overburdened with toxins causing the toxins to leak into the circulation, which can deposit elsewhere in the body. If it is carried to the brain, it can cause neurological problems like Parkinson's disease and multiple sclerosis.

Patients with high toxic burden will usually need to undergo chelation to enhance the excretion of the heavy metals out from the body. Once chelation occurs, the patient would be prescribed binders to pull out the heavy metals from the stools to be excreted.

Colonics would be useful in patients who are usually constipated to enhance the excretion of toxins out from the body via the stools. (see below on Colonics)

The next step is to treat the patient's "leaky gut" by treating any underlying gut dysbiosis and infections and avoiding food allergy triggers that may cause inflammation of the gut wall. Short chain fatty acids like Butyrate and Ghee are healing to the gut wall and bone broth containing glutamine helps in the repair of the gut wall. Additional supplements containing glutamine and aloe would be useful to heal the gut wall.

COLONICS

A colonic is a method of irrigating your colon by pumping the colon with warm water and flushing it out repeatedly. It sends water up the colon using pressure and then water comes out continuously like in a closed system.

The colon is the last part of our digestive system where water and minerals get absorbed from our food into our circulation. This is also where most of the remaining foods are eliminated. The colon also eliminates unwanted debris from our circulation eliminated with the faces. The colon houses a myriad of bacteria and it is this intestinal floral that helps in detoxification, digestion and regulating our immune system. Having a healthy gut also helps in regulating a healthy mood since most of our serotonin receptors lie in the gut.

Sometimes during a colon cleanse, a thick gooey material can come out, and this is called the mucoid plaque, which has accumulated in the colon over time and blocking proper elimination of the waste from our body.

An enema is different in that water is pumped in then interrupted to let the water come out by gravity. The water doesn't go as high up the colon as compared to doing a colonic.

Colonics should be done only during a cleansing program and not too regularly as it may alter the intestinal flora and in worse cases, in people with inflammatory bowels or diverticulitis, it may lead to colon perforation. So, it should only be performed by trained therapists.

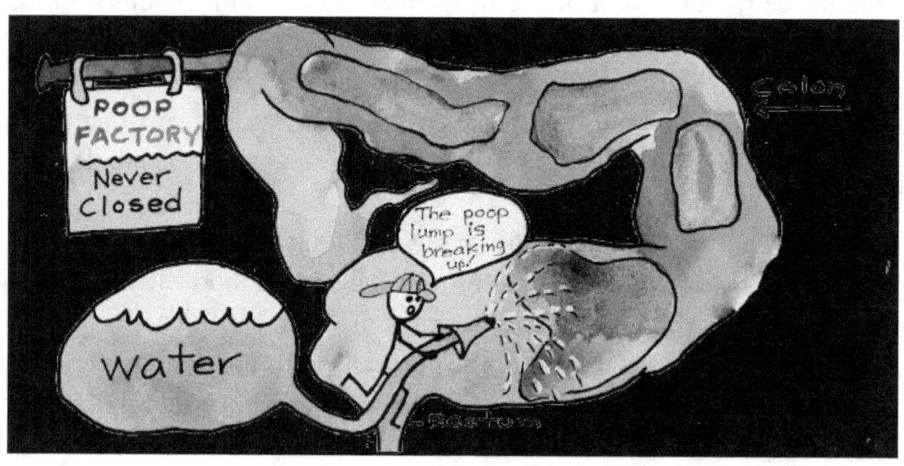

CHAPTER 7B

Brain and nervous system symptoms and toxicity

Toxic metals exposure has been linked to developing neurodegenerative disease in humans. These toxic metals like Cadmium (Cd), lead (Pb), arsenic (As), mercury (Hg) and Thallium (Th) cross the blood-brain barrier to enter into the brain. Long-term accumulation of these toxic metals in the brain leads to developing neurodegenerative diseases.

Many metals like iron, chromium, at trace levels are essential for life, but excess levels can be toxic to the cells. Neurodegenerative disease is one of the most common manifestations of metal toxicity. Heavy metals have been linked to neurological disorders like Alzheimer's Disease (AD), Parkinson's Disease (PD), Amyotrophic Lateral Sclerosis (ALS) and Multiple Sclerosis (MS).

Both environmental and genetic factors are responsible for the accumulation of heavy metals, causing neurological conditions. Environmental factors include ingestion of food and water containing heavy metal contaminants, occupational heavy metals exposure, etc. There is a high incidence of neurodegenerative diseases, for example, ALS, PD and AD linked to workers working in the automobile and paint industries where there is a high exposure of these employees to metals used in the factories. (3)

Various genetic factors predispose the body to accumulate heavy metals. Patients with methylation gene defects can lead to poor methylation and issues with detoxification of heavy metals. MTHFR C677 T allele SNP was shown to alter biochemical pathways in folate metabolism. TT homozygotes are more sensitive to heavy metals and

59

other environmental toxins. A well down genetic disease, Wilson's disease, is an autosomal recessive disorder due to the mutation of the ATP7B gene, which encodes the copper transporter leading to the accumulation of copper in the liver and brain.

Excess accumulation of metals could lead to cell toxicity and pathological damage to the function of the cells. These metal ions could change the membrane potential, particularly the neutrons, and can also affect the activity of proteins, enzymes and nucleic acids, which can cause cell toxicity. They can also help to generate ROS (reactive oxide species), which can cause oxidative damage to the cells. Many heavy metals like cadmium and lead are highly oxidative and highly toxic. They can cause membrane depolarization by blocking calcium influx and causing cell death. (4) In the normal brain, metal homeostasis is tightly regulated by carrier proteins (e.g., Ferritin, transferrin, ceruloplasmin). These stored metals are only released during metabolic needs. However, excess metal accumulation can occur when there is abnormal sequestration of the metals. This can lead to losing the homeostatic balance and loss of the regulation of the metals across the cell membranes. For example, in Alzheimer's disease, iron and copper are found in increased levels in the brain. (5) In Parkinson's disease, there is an increase in iron and a decrease in zinc. (6) There are numerous scientific studies that link trace metal accumulations to Alzheimer-type mental deterioration. A team of researchers from the National Institute of Neurological and Communicative Disorders and Stroke (NINCDS) found a high accumulation of aluminum in the brains of the natives of Guan who had died either from Amyotrophic lateral sclerosis (ALS) or Parkinsonism dementia. Similarly, Dr Daniel P. Perl of the University of Vermont has found abnormal levels of aluminum accumulated within the neurofibrillary tangles found in the brain cells of patients with Alzheimer's disease.

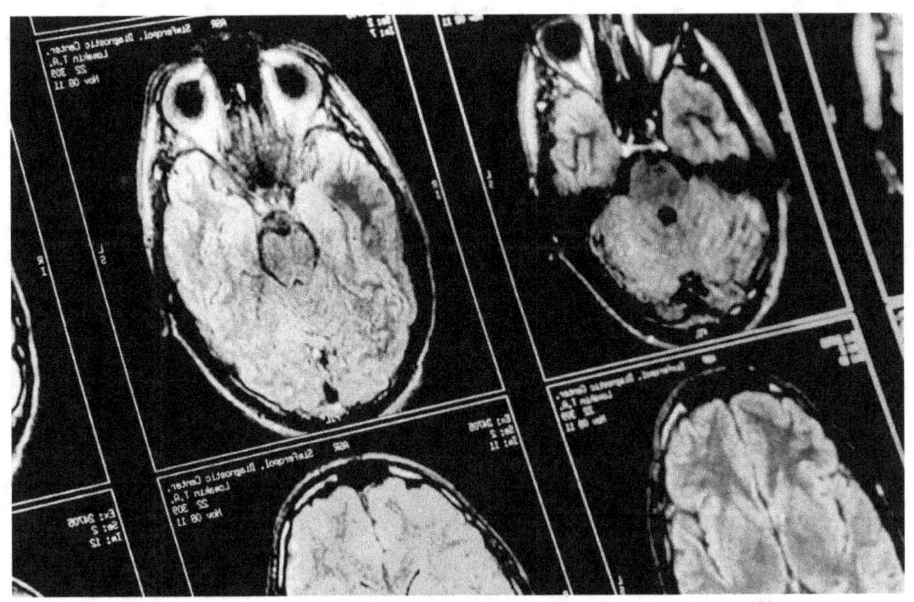

How do toxic substances get into our body?

Toxins enter our bodies via several channels, including through our food, our drinking water and from pollution in the air we breathe in and even through our skin transdermally.

These toxins are carried into our liver whereby they undergo phase I and II detoxification reactions so that can be removed from our body. However, if our body system cannot remove them, they are carried by the bloodstream all over our body. They become more harmful and can cause oxidative damage in our bodies.

How toxins get into our brain?

Our brain is protected by a membrane called the Blood-Brain Barrier, which protects the brain and the spine from toxic substances. The BBB allows certain lipid soluble compounds to pass through. Some of these toxic substances cross the BBB and deposit in the brain, causing neurotoxic symptoms. Some of these toxic substances include lipid soluble pesticides, and heavy metals like lead. Toxic metals can affect the brain in these ways:

- Weakening of the blood-brain barrier
- Interfering with the levels of the neurotransmitters causing changes in level of dopamine, serotonin, norepinephrine, etc.

- Damage to the myelin sheath of the nerve cells causing demyelination
- Increase in free radicals and oxidative stress

Lead toxicity to the brain

Lead exposure has been linked to low IQ, aggressive behavior, criminal activity and neurodegenerative diseases.

The neurotoxic effects of lead are linked to apoptosis (cell death), affecting the neurotransmitter storage and release and causing changes to neurotransmitter receptors, mitochondria, astroglia and oligodendroglia cells. Acute toxicity may present as immediate symptoms, but chronic lead toxicity may cause delayed reactions, including loss of memory, visions, cognitive and behavioral problems, and brain damage and mental retardation. High lead exposures have been linked to neuropsychological issues like anti-social behaviors, delinquency, and violence.

In children, exposure in Utero, in infancy or in early childhood can lead to issues like brain damage / mental retardation, behavioral problems, low IQ, hearing loss, hyperactivity, developmental delays, behavioral problems, poor school performance, or even attention deficit hyperactivity disorder (ADHD). Young children are especially sensitive to heavy metals due to their immature blood-brain barrier allowing the toxins to pass through more easily to the brain and interfering with developing their brain cells. For example, lead toxicity can affect the IQ and brain development in young children but may have little effect on the mental capacity of the adult. (7)

Neurotoxicity of Copper and Zinc

Excess copper can have a significant neurologic consequence well described in Wilson's disease, a genetic disorder that causes a build-up of copper, leading to neurobehavioral changes similar to schizophrenia. Excess brain copper is also a common finding in neurodegenerative diseases like Alzheimer's disease.

Zinc deficiency has adverse effects on neurodevelopment. On the other hand, excess zinc is also linked to neurodegenerative disease. (8) Excess zinc has been linked to neuronal injury observed in cerebral ischemia, epilepsy and brain trauma. The neurotoxicity effects of zinc stems from mitochondrial production of reactive oxygen species and disrupting metabolic enzymes leading to the activation of apoptotic processes. Zinc's role in Alzheimer's disease has also been linked to excess zinc triggering beta-amyloid aggregation and neuronal plaque formation.

Heavy metals and neurodegenerative diseases

Complex neurological problems can be caused not only by mercury but also with the presence of other heavy metals. There are usually striking connections between neurological problems with amalgams and root canal treatments. It is likely that galvanic currents created by the metals in root canals and amalgams release highly toxic metals in their organic form, and toxic thioether and xylols.

There are numerous papers that have shown that heavy metals like aluminum, mercury and other toxic metals have been linked to the development of Alzheimer's disease. (9) For mercury, there has been published data showing a positive relation between mercury exposure and the risk of Alzheimer's disease. One of the causative factors is that mercury increases oxidative stress. Mercury exposure is mainly from fish consumption, dental amalgams or vaccines containing mercury. Canadian investigators have found aluminum at exceptionally high levels in the brains of some Alzheimer's patients. The accumulation of toxic metals may impair enzyme reactions and block metabolic pathways and hence accelerate the development of neurodegenerative diseases.

Parkinson's disease

For Parkinson's disease, it has been linked to metal exposures, including iron, mercury, manganese and lead. (10) Research has shown elevated iron levels in the Substantia Nigra of Parkinson's disease patients. These metals appear to increase the formation of mitochondria reactive species (ROS). Mitochondria dysfunction leads to biochemical events, which includes the formation of reactive oxygen species (ROS) and the reduction in the production of dopamine. A combination of increased ROS and reactive iron ions leads to developing neurotransmitter dysfunction.

There have been several reports of patients with Parkinson's disease where high levels of mercury intoxication had been demonstrated, and these cases usually improve or stabilize once the amalgam source had been removed with detoxification given. Unfortunately, in many of these patients, lasting damage had been done to the dopamine processing and would still need to take their dopamine medication, but clinically they felt better with slowing down the progression of their disease.

Multiple sclerosis

MS is a multifactorial and multi toxic disease, a large part of it originating from amalgams in the teeth. Thus, an important part of treatment is cleansing or removing amalgams or root canal fillings from the teeth.

In a study carried out at the University of Lexington, histochemical samples were taken from degenerated myelin sheath of MS lesions and examined electrophoretically together with tissue from root apex and pulp of root canal treated teeth. It was shown from this study that toxic proteins in both cases were the same.

Toxicity causing depression

Toxic chemical poisoning can cause a chemical imbalance in the brain leading to symptoms of depression. Most of the cases involve lead, mercury, cadmium or arsenic. (11) This form of depression is estimated to affect 5% of the depressive patient population.

Common symptoms of the toxicity caused depression includes:

- Depression that suddenly arise from a previously well person
- Frequent abdominal pain
- Associated headaches and body aches
- Chronic fatigue
- Brain fog
- Failure to respond well to antidepressants

If the patient presents with the above symptoms and has a likelihood of exposure to heavy metals, the doctor can prescribe certain tests like the hair toxic metals test or the oral DMSA urine challenge test to look for high levels of toxic metals as a possible cause for the depressive symptoms.

Treatment involves proper chelation to remove lead and other heavy metals and supplementation with nutrients like calcium and zinc and antioxidants usually produce significant benefits and good results.

Multiple Chemical Sensitivity and Toxicity

Multiple Chemical Sensitivity is a condition whereby the patient develops multiple symptoms triggered by multiple environmental chemicals, foods and drugs, and can is disabling. The diagnosis is controversial as there is lack of evidence and research linking environmental agents with symptoms. Treatment of the symptoms by avoidance of the environmental chemicals, dietary change, detoxification may help to alleviate the symptoms.

Symptoms

The most common complaints are vague symptoms like fatigue, malaise, brain fog, bodily pains, etc., but usually, the patient can present the history of these symptoms being linked to certain chemical triggers. The usual symptom provoking chemicals usually emit some smell or fragrances like perfumes, paints, cleaning solvents, etc.

Unlike allergies to food and medicines, whereby an immunological reaction triggers an objective physical reaction like rash or swelling, intolerance in MCS is subjective. They can have subjective reactions to multiple foods and medications that do not correspond to an allergic response. Laboratory testing may reveal no abnormalities. Even doing immunological tests may show up as normal.

Pathogenesis

Many controversies surround what is the pathology of MCS. Some postulate it is caused by an overwhelming toxic damage to the immune system from environmental chemicals, foods and drugs. The lack of objective evidence distinguishes these groups of patients from those suffering from multiple allergies, autoimmune diseases or diseases associated with immunodeficiencies.

One theory proposes that patients suffering from MCS fail to detoxify environmental chemicals due to a defect of detoxification genes and enzymes triggered by vitamins and minerals deficiencies. It is believed these patients with MCS carry a high body burden of environmental toxicants and xenobiotic chemicals which they cannot detoxify from their body.

Diagnosis

The diagnostic work-up includes measuring the components of the immune system such as circulating immunoglobulins, presence of autoantibodies, and measuring lymphocytes with surface markers. It may help to check the detoxification genes and also measuring the organic pollutant level and doing the urine heavy metal challenge test to look for chemical and toxic metal triggers. Also, checking for vitamin and minerals may help to optimize the detoxification process.

Treatment

The primary form of treatment and the most effective would be the avoidance of the environmental chemicals.

Working on the diet, for example, the Elimination Diet, helps to eliminate certain foods that may trigger an unknown sensitive reaction. It may help to do a food sensitivity test to have an objective list of foods to avoid in the diet to avoid further triggering an overactive immune system.

Optimizing vitamins and minerals lacking help to boost the immune system and also strengthen the detoxification pathways.

Starting a regimen of detoxification, including oral supplements, binders, infra-red sauna, colonics and liver enzymes-stimulating herbs may help to boost the body's detoxification system to remove chemicals and heavy metals from the body.

Working on the home environment is crucial when you are suffering from MCS. Clean up your existing house and replace the toxic house agents like cleaners and shampoos with safer alternatives. In serious cases, it may involve packing and moving into a less toxic home environment. Some of the toxic building materials include glues, carpet, paint, wood preservatives, and insulation. Remember when moving or building a new home these potential exposures you may have and to try to minimize them:

1) Mold
Some studies have found that up to fifty percent of all homes have mold growth in some ways. Especially in Hong Kong where you have moisture and high humidity, there is a conducive environment for mold to thrive.

2) Lead-based paint
Lead is a heavy metal material that can build up toxic levels with repeated exposure. It was 1978 that lead paint was banned and many homes built before that have walls that contain lead paint.

3) Volatile Organic Compounds (VOCs)
VOCs are gases that escape from materials such as body shampoos, cleaning solvents, plastics, furniture and building materials, etc. These chemicals, when inhaled into the body, can induce chemical sensitivity and increase the risk of cancer.

When our homes are sealed up tight for air-conditioning, this can lead to a build-up of polluted indoor air and this can further worsen the symptoms of MCS. Thus, it is essential to have an air purifier that can help remove many of these pollutants from our air. Also, choose natural cleaning and body products to minimize your exposure to VOCs and xenoestrogens.

Methylation and detoxification
Methylation is a biochemical process whereby a methyl group is added to a molecule. Methylation can change the activity of a DNA segment without changing the sequence. When located in a gene promoter, DNA methylation typically acts to repress gene transcription.

Methylation is important for many biochemical reactions in the body, one of which is to methylate and prevent the overactivity of neurotransmitters and the other is to create glutathione [M1] through the CBS pathway to enable the body to detoxify and prevent the build-up of toxins and free radicals. Methylation needs to be addressed early in patients with signs of toxicity or multiple chemical sensitivity.

Patients presenting with the MTHFR mutation have a defective MTHFR enzyme. They produce 30 to 70% less methyl-folate than someone without the mutation does and this can affect the detoxification pathway.

Impaired methylation can lead to depression, anxiety, histamine intolerance, increased risk of cancer, hormone imbalance, poor detox capacity, infertility, birth defects, fatigue, and low energy.

The Methylation Cycle

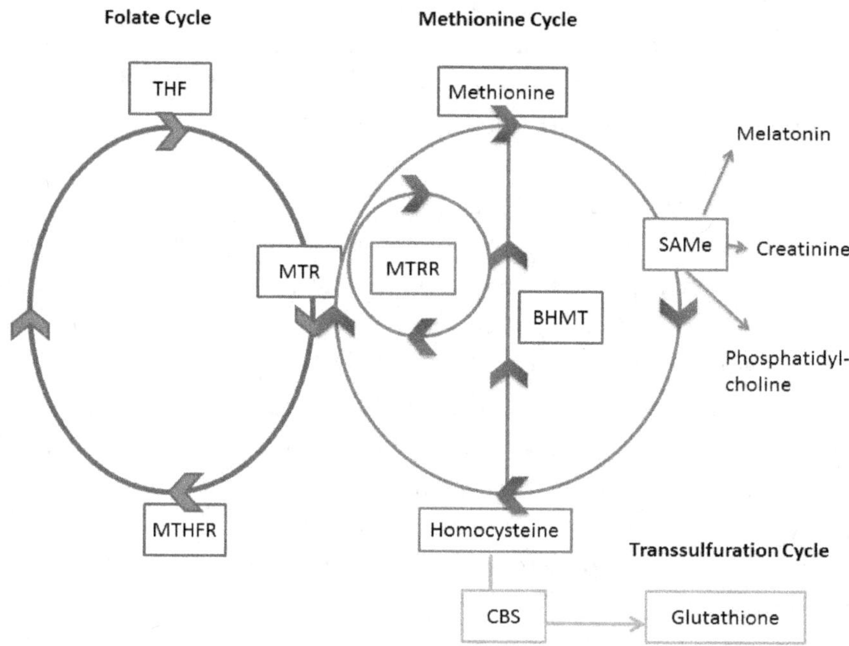

A few natural ways to support this cycle are:
1. Have adequate nutrients - The two most important nutrients in methylation pathways are B12 and folate, but other nutrients such as methionine, cysteine, taurine, DHA, zinc, magnesium, potassium, riboflavin, niacin, pyridoxine, betaine, choline, and sulfur also play a role. Inadequate intake of any of these nutrients can impair methylation. Foods high in these methylation-supporting nutrients include beets, spinach, mushrooms, eggs, organ meats, and shellfish.
2. Eat foods high in natural folate.
3. Support your body's natural detoxification process through

infrared saunas, IV glutathione, exercise, healthy foods, and chelation supplements.

4. Remove mold from your home.
5. Avoid toxins.
6. Manage your stress.
7. Support good gut health.

Allergies and Skin Manifestations of Toxicity

Allergy or skin rashes represent the immune system's excessive reaction to an allergen, normally due to disrupting the body's internal milieu. Stress very often can also worsen the allergy or skin rash. Avoiding the allergens, be it inhalant or food allergen, is only part of the solution. One must look at the underlying cause in the body creating the overactive immune system.

Functional investigations to look at triggering factors for the allergies:
- Food and inhalant allergy tests - for gE, IgG, and IgG4
- Total IgE and histamine
- Comprehensive stool analysis to look at gut dysbiosis, leaky gut and inflammation
- Urine heavy metal challenge test - in allergies we often find a high level of aluminium, lead and mercury intoxication.
- Nutrient evaluation test - In allergic patients, we often see a reduced zinc and selenium level with high levels of phosphorus, magnesium and calcium (due to over-acidity of the tissues).

Factors favouring allergies and skin manifestations
- An over acidic milieu causes the mast cells to react with greater sensitivity. Thu in treating an allergic patient, it is important to create an alkaline milieu using alkaline powders and changing the diet to include more alkaline foods (more vegetables, fruits, potatoes, avocados, chestnuts).

- Avoid foods high in histamines - meat, fish and shellfish and tomatoes.
- Avoid animal proteins - especially dairy products, pork, fish and eggs.
- Poor intestinal flora and dysbiosis creating intestinal permeability
- Heavy metals toxicity
- Vaccination - vaccines contain mercury which frequently trigger allergies. There have been many reports of children developing eczema after the vaccinations.
- Mould and Candida - most people with allergies suffer primarily from mould toxicity. Besides allergies, they frequently present with tiredness, recurrent infections, low mood, vision problems, etc. Candida is frequently linked to allergies. However, the treatment should not be to use antifungals to treat the Candida, which will further disrupt the intestinal flora; rather, it should be to treat the underlying heavy metal toxicity or gut dysbiosis.

Common symptoms associated with overexposure to heavy metals

An unhealthy accumulation of heavy metals can disrupt the body's balance and lead to a myriad of symptoms, including chronic fatigue, depression, anxiety, insomnia, digestive problems, skin issues and even autoimmune disease.

Heavy metals can disrupt our body's biology in a few ways. They cause cell damage to the mitochondria, they can disrupt multiple enzyme functions, they can disrupt our hormonal balance, they can also lead to disruption of gut microbiome causing gut leafiness, and stimulating the immune system to become over-reactive.

Chronic low-level metal toxicity commonly is under diagnosed as either a proper history is not taken, or the physician is unaware of such a diagnosis. Left untreated, it can lead to a myriad of symptoms, including fatigue, depression, insomnia, skin issues, digestive disorders, etc. Removing exposure to the source of the Heavy Metals and boosting the body's innate ability for detoxification is important to help alleviate the symptoms for the patient.

Steps to take include:

1. Remove your exposure to heavy metals. A common source of heavy metals I have seen is dental mercury amalgams. Check your mouth if you have any metal fillings and go to a biological dentist to remove the mercury fillings.

2. Increase intake of foods that help in detoxification, including cruciferous vegetables, onions, garlic, green tea and cilantro.

3. Increase fibre intake as fibre acts like a binder to help bind heavy metals out from the body. High fibre foods include flaxseeds, legumes, vegetables, brown rice, quinoa. I would also recommend taking supplements in the form of psyllium husk a few times a day to increase fibre in the diet.

4. Consume high-quality proteins like organic grass-fed beef, grass-fed lamb, etc., as these sources of proteins contain essential amino acids to help in phase II detoxification of the liver.

5. Optimize intake of minerals either through foods or supplement forms, including Selenium, Iron, Zinc, B vitamins, Vitamin C and all the B vitamins essential for boosting Phase I detoxification in the liver.

6. Increase intake of phytonutrients and antioxidants in the diet to boost the antioxidant level in the body to fight free radicals caused by the heavy metals in the body. Have a high intake of colourful vegetables high in phytonutrients, and also increase intake of alpha-lipoic acid, N-acetyl-cysteine and glutathione for antioxidation.

For less severe exposure, more gentle methods could support detoxification, which include taking glutathione supplements, NAC, ALA, B vitamins, vitamin C, selenium or zinc. Add on natural binders like zeolite, charcoal, silica or cholestyramine to help bind these heavy metals when removed by the liver after the deterioration process.

CHAPTER 8

Detoxification Food Plans

The definition of detoxification is "the body's physiological process of rendering chemicals, compounds, hormones, and toxicants less harmful", also termed metabolic detoxification. The body eliminates toxins and wastes from the body through the liver, kidneys, large intestine, lymphatic and sweat glands.

We have all been through times when our body feels like it has been overloaded - from stress, from food and from toxins in our environment. It can manifest as abdominal bloating and irregular bowels, or even on the skin with acne, unexplained rashes from sensitivity, or vague symptoms like low energy and brain fog. Usually, it happens after we travelled to other countries and we overindulged, or after a holiday season like Christmas during which we feasted excessively on rich foods when we are with friends and family. Your body needs some time off sometimes and it is a good habit to do a cleansing detox every 3-6months regularly just to reset your system and let your liver rest to move waste and toxins out of your body. Once your liver rests and reset, your detoxification process will work better, and your metabolism will reset itself.

Sometimes, our body cannot clear toxins and they accumulate in our body, causing symptoms like body aches, fatigue, brain fog, etc. The reasons could be increased exposure to toxins, constipation, eating a poor nutrient diet, overloading your body with alcohol and ingestion of foods high in hormones and pesticides, being under stress, and having a lack of sleep. A person could also genetically not detoxify well and hence will be more prone to heavy metals and pollutants accumulating in the body. The principles of the Detox Food Plan are to:

I) Eliminate common food triggers

II) Focus on nutrients that enhance the function of the gut and liver to support detoxification and elimination.

III) Reduce acidity of the body and enhance alkalization.

IV) Enhance elimination through the kidneys by frequent ingestion of water and detox tea.

Detoxification can best be done through a 3-day intense vegetable or juice cleanse, a 7-day cleansing elimination diet, or a month-long clean eating plan.

I) Elimination of food triggers

During detox, the main foods we need to eliminate from our diet, preferably for at least 4 weeks are:

- coffee
- alcohol
- dairy products from cow's milk
- gluten
- corn
- nightshade vegetables (tomatoes, eggplants, peppers, potatoes)
- refined sugar and carbs
- shellfish
- white rice and white bread
- eggs
- soy
- fish high in mercury

These foods are usually inflammatory in nature and they are best avoided during detoxification. The aim of detoxification is to allow your body's organs of detoxification to work more efficiently to reduce the body burden or toxic load of chemicals - these organs of elimination include the liver, kidneys, large intestine, lymphatic system, and sweat glands.

The food plan also emphasizes strict restriction of foods high in toxins by encouraging as best as possible intake of organic, seasonal foods not genetically modified. Also, to take clean lean animal proteins or wild caught fish rather than farmed fish.

Ways to avoid intake of harmful food substances:
- Choose lean meats over fatty meats as pesticides accumulate in fats.
- Eat organic animal and vegetable produce where possible.
- Peeling off the outer skin of fruits and vegetables before ingestion
- Avoid foods in the "Dirty Dozen" which are high in pesticide residues and eat more from the "Clean 15" (foods low in pesticides). (Check the Environmental Working Group for the list of foods)
- Avoid foods with preservatives, additional food colorings or with artificial sweeteners.
- Reduce eating canned foods or foods packed in plastic containers, which can contain xenoestrogens that disrupt the endocrine function of the body.
- Cook using non-toxic pans and pots.
- Ensure that drinking water is filtered, and put a filter on the showerhead.

II) Foods and nutrients to enhance detoxification through the liver and gut

Think of the liver as the main hub of the detoxification process. With our poor diet and lifestyle, stress and lack of sleep, the liver becomes clogged up and overburdened with toxic load and hence becomes sluggish, resulting in also poor metabolism and issues like weight gain and fatty liver. The aim of the Detox Food Plan is to unclog the liver, maximize nutrient intake to stimulate the detox liver enzymes and ensure proper detoxification. The gut is the next step after the liver conjugates the toxin to eliminate the toxin through the gut. Hence maintaining good bowel movements and good gut health is also a key step in detoxification.

Various nutrients are required to fuel the liver's phase I and phase II detoxification. Especially for patients with polymorphism of the genetic SNP for cytochrome P450 that affects the phase I detoxification, eating a nutrient-dense diet to improve phase I and II liver conjugation would be useful. Plant foods especially from the cruciferous family (broccoli, Brussels sprouts, cabbage, cauliflower, watercress) and other vegetables rich in B vitamins (spinach, sweet potato, lentils, beans) and flavonoids (blueberries, raspberries, strawberries, parsley and all colorful fruits and vegetables) help improve both phase I and II on liver detoxification. High-quality lean animal or plant protein helps to facilitate more phase II conjugation. Intake of foods with high antioxidant properties helps protect against overproduction of phase I metabolites, which can sometimes produce reactive oxygen intermediates and free radicals and cause tissue damage. The foods include those high in Vitamin A, C and E, selenium, thiols containing foods like garlic and onions, and foods high in polyphenols and flavonoids (berries, cherries, etc). (18)

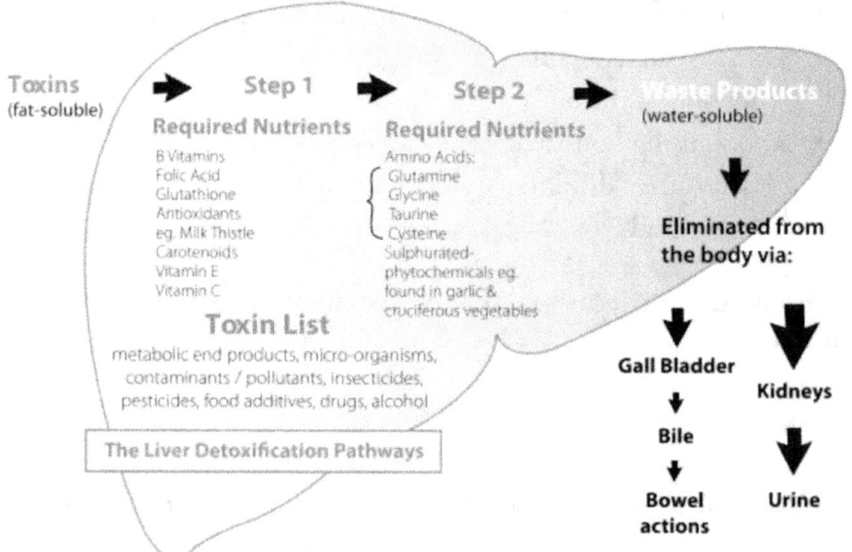

III) Reduce acidity and enhancing alkalinity through the diet

The typical modern-day diet contains a high level of acidifying foods like animal proteins, wheat, gluten, dairy and refined or processed sugars. This could lead to increased dietary acid load and disrupt the acid-alkali homeostasis in the body, eventually resulting in chronic diseases like arthritis, eczema, kidney stones, high blood pressure, etc. Doing an alkaline-based detox could lead to more effective excretion of toxins from the body. The body's pH level is considered healthy if pH level is 7.0 or above. The rule is to eat a diet 80% alkaline-forming foods and 20% acid-forming foods to maintain a good pH balance. When our body's pH is too acidic, the body will work to balance the pH by releasing alkaline-rich minerals like calcium, phosphorus and magnesium from the bones, teeth and organs into the bloodstream. These minerals, once pulled out, can lead to a weaker immune system, general fatigue and body aches and vulnerability to bacteria and viruses and even cancer cells.

List of alkaline-forming foods:
- most fruits and vegetables
- nuts and seeds
- herbal teas
- green juice
- lemon in water
- chia seeds

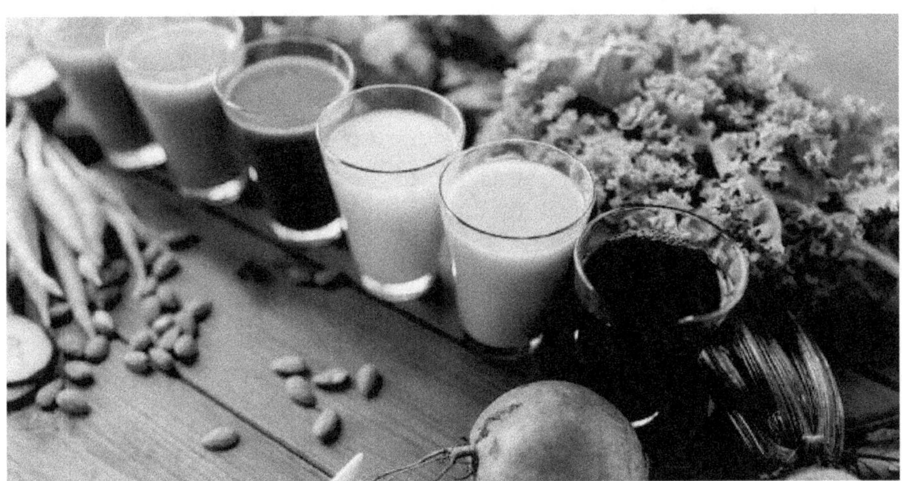

List of acid-forming foods to avoid
- most grains
- meats
- dairy products
- processed foods
- rancid oils
- refined sugars
- coffee
- alcohol

Cells with a healthy pH can effectively absorb nutrients and minerals they require and eliminate the waste products. If the pH is imbalanced, the cells become weakened and their ability to repair and rejuvenate is also inhibited, which can also lead to premature aging of the cells. An alkaline diet will help to maintain healthy cells and rid them of toxins while boosting the body's immune system to fight infections and also cancer cells.

IV) Encouraging healthy elimination through the stools and urine

After the liver conjugates the toxins into metabolites after phase I conjugation, the metabolites could become more toxic if they are not properly processed through the phase II conjugation. Antioxidants are required to protect the body from these reactive metabolites. After phase II conjugation, they are then excreted through the stools and the urine. So, a focus of the detox food plan is also to enhance elimination besides conjugation by ingesting more fiber-rich foods to enhance stool elimination. Drinking more water, green tea and detox tea throughout the day helps to ensure the elimination of the toxins through the kidneys.

Principles of the detox diet based on biological principles

The biological method of detoxification works on maintaining a balance in the body's milieu. The benefits that a person can obtain from following this detox diet is firstly to detoxify the body and ease the toxic burden on the liver to enable the liver to function better to process detoxification and also enable the metabolic processes to run smoothly in the body.

Another goal of this diet is to de-acidify the body's internal environment as too much acidity in the body can lead to issues like inflammation causing arthritis, body aches, fatigue, etc. The third principle after detoxifying and de-acidifying is to balance and maintain healthy intestinal flora. The gut is the main organ in the body responsible for our immune system as it contains 70% of the body's immune system and also serotonin receptors responsible for maintaining our mood. Maintaining a healthy gut flora will help us to achieve an optimal immune system to fight diseases and also maintain the optimal mood. But if our gut is not healthy and is "leaky", it can trigger autoimmune reactions and lead to issues like allergies, make us susceptible to frequent infections and lead to mood issues like depression and anxiety.

This diet can be done for a month once every 3-6 months to reset and detoxify the body, then we can go back to our normal diet and lifestyle. This way, our body may frequently reboot from too many toxins in our diet and environment, thus preventing toxic pollutants and heavy metals to accumulate in our body, causing harmful effects. For busy people like us who indulge in rich foods and travel frequently with unhealthy diets and lifestyle, it is important to reboot the system frequently to enable the liver to work better for our metabolism. Just like a computer system, when we open up too many programs on our computer, after some time, the computer will hang as it is overworked. Sometimes, we need to switch the computer off and reboot the system again so it will run smoothly and process things at a faster speed. This same principle works for our body system.

Benefits of the diet:
- Detoxifies the body
- De-acidifies the internal environment
- Develops a proper intestinal flora

Rules of the detox diet

The first week of the diet is completely vegan. The diet consists mostly of fresh vegetables with small amounts of fruit and very little grain with minimal gluten.

In the second and third weeks, add a very modest portion of proteins with some goat and sheep cheese, legumes and more whole grains are included.

Finally in the fourth week, add a modest amount of protein from clean, lean meat like organic hormone chicken and turkey, clean fish and organic grass-fed beef with some whole grains.

We can further increase the nutritional value of the vegetables we ingest by using healthy dressings. Dress the vegetables with at least 1 tbsp of fresh lemon juice and extra virgin olive oil or flaxseed oil, and sprinkle sunflower seeds, pumpkin seeds or flaxseeds over your salads.

Include a small amount of goat and sheep cheese or yoghurt during weeks two and three will provide some added proteins to the body, which is also important in supporting phase II conjugation process of the liver. Some principles to follow for the detox diet:

- At lunch, you should have both raw and cooked vegetables but at night, eat only cooked vegetables only.
- No fruit should be eaten after 4 pm. It ferments in the gut at night and stresses the liver.
- Do not skip mid-morning and afternoon snacks - crucial to maintain blood sugar level.
- Drink at least 3L of herbal tea and purified water a day.
- Begin your day with a piece of lemon in warm water or a spoonful of apple cider vinegar to alkalize the body.
- Have a bowl of vegetable alkaline broth daily
- Take 1 tbsp of pure flaxseed oil or extra virgin coconut oil every morning with breakfast.

For a total detox diet

- Vegetables make up the bulk of the diet for the whole month.
- No coffee, caffeinated beverage, sugar, meat, wheat products, dairy products, or alcohol is allowed.
- Restrict to herbal teas and alkaline soup or broth.
- Use a modest amount of Himalayan salt in the cooking.

Example of the Detox Diet

I)   WEEK ONE

Breakfast

- 1 bowl of alkaline broth
- 1/2 cup fresh grapefruit juice
- 1 tbsp pure extra virgin coconut oil (you can put it in the oats)
- 1/4 cup steel-cut oats cooked in 1 cup water with 1 date until very soft; no other sweetener
- 1 small apple or 1/2 avocado dressed with 1 tbsp fresh lemon juice and 1 tsp extra virgin olive oil
- 1 cup decaffeinated green tea or herb tea

Mid-morning snack

- 1/2 apple or 1 small carrot

Lunch

- SALAD: shredded raw vegetables or steamed vegetables dressed with lemon juice and extra virgin olive oil or flaxseed oil. Sprinkle with sunflower seeds, pumpkin seeds or flaxseeds or add good nuts like crushed almond nuts and macadamia nuts.

Dinner

- Steamed vegetable plate: broccoli floret, sliced carrots, 1 small gold potato, sliced and all lightly steamed. Do not overcook. May splash with 2 tsp lemon juice or balsamic vinegar and extra virgin olive oil. Sprinkle with 1 tbsp sunflower seeds.

II) WEEK TWO AND WEEK THREE

- Maintain an alkaline balance but gradually incorporate small amounts of whole grains and goat and sheep dairy to vary your diet. Embellish your salad with a light sprinkling of sunflower seeds, pumpkin seeds or flaxseeds.
- Drink at least 3 L of purified water, unsweetened herbal tea and alkalinizing broth.
- Begin your day with a piece of lemon in warm water or a spoonful of apple cider vinegar to alkalinize the body.
- Take 1 tbsp of pure flaxseed oil or extra virgin coconut oil every morning with breakfast.

Breakfast

- 1 bowl of vegetable alkaline broth (can be prepared the night before and heat up)
- 1/2 cup grapefruit juice
- 1 tbsp flaxseed oil or extra virgin coconut oil (can be added into oats)
- 1/2 cup steel oats cooked in 1 cup water with 1 date cook till very soft.
- 1 small banana or 1/2 cup dried fruit compote
- 1 splice of spelt bread toasted with 1/2 tsp butter and 2 tsp natural sweetened fruit preserves
- 1 cup green tea or herb tea

Mid-morning

- 1/2 avocado with a squeeze of lemon juice or 1/2 an apple or some carrot sticks

Lunch

- Your choice of shredded raw vegetables dressed with lemon juice and extra virgin olive oil sprinkle with sunflower seeds, pumpkin seeds or flaxseeds or add good nuts like crushed almond nuts and macadamia nuts.
- 2 rye crisps

- Steamed vegetable plate: broccoli florets, sliced carrots, 1 small Yukon potato sliced and lightly steamed. May splash with 2 tbsp of lemon juice or balsamic vinegar and extra virgin olive oil. Sprinkle with 1 tbsp sunflower seeds.

Mid-afternoon snack
- A small container of goat or sheep yoghurt
- Or 1 rye crisp with sweet potato pine nut spread

Supper
- 1/2 cup fresh carrot or vegetable juice
- 1 bowl of alkaline soup broth
- 1/2 cup olive oil steamed spinach
- Twice-baked potato with some blue cheese and broccoli
- Cup of peppermint herb tea
- Can add some whole grains like quinoa or can have 1/3 cup cooked basmati rice with 1/3 cup marinated roast beets.

III) WEEK FOUR

For the fourth week of the detox diet, follow the above principle for week two and week three but add in a portion of proteins from clean, lean organic meat once a day for the added protein intake.

CHAPTER 9

Detoxification Recipes

10 healthy recipes to be included in the Detox Diet
Here we have included 10 detox recipes for sharing some food ideas you can include that are good for detoxifying your body.
1. Alkaline broth
2. Sweet potato, carrot ginger chowder
3. Sweet pea soup with fresh mint
4. Sweet potato, kale, cauliflower and onions gratin
5. Black bean burger with cashews and carrots
6. Lentil and pumpkin soup
7. Asian sesame slaw
8. Healthy chicken soup with lentils
9. Pecan crusted catfish with pineapple slaw
10. Red lentil coconut curry with organic chicken

1. Alkaline broth recipe

This is the basis of the alkaline broth with the function of alkalinising the body for optimising detoxification every day.

Makes about 7 cups broth; 31/2 cups vegetables

Ingredients
- 1 1/2 cup zucchini
- 1 cup cut green beans
- 1 cup celery diced
- 1 cup diced carrots
- sea salt (optional)

Method
1. Put all the vegetables in a large saucepan with 8 cups of filtered water/non-chlorinated spring water. Bring to a boil and skim off any scum that rises to the top.
2. Once boiled, reduce it to a simmer and cook the vegetables for another 15 minutes until soft. You can add in the optional sea salt.
3. Remove from the heat and let it stand covered for about 10 minutes and serve as directed.
4. Keep the remaining broth about 2 days in the refrigerator and the remaining in the freezer and in individual measured containers.
5. The vegetables may be eaten the first 2 days, and any remaining should not be frozen but should be discarded.

2. Sweet potato carrot ginger chowder

Sweet potato is packed with lots of nutrients and they are an excellent source of beta carotene, vitamin C and potassium, and is a rich source of fiber. Adding a bit of turmeric powder seasoning with fresh ginger gives a spicy touch to this soup, which helps improve digestion and reduce inflammation.

This soup can be prepared and consumed in 2 days.

For 4-6 servings

Ingredients
- 2 tbsp extra virgin olive oil
- 1/4 cup sliced white leeks
- 2 tsp fresh minced ginger
- 5 medium carrots, peeled and thinly sliced
- 1 tsp turmeric powder and 1 tsp ground cumin
- 6 cups of organic vegetable or chicken broth
- some sea salt for seasoning
- 2 medium-size sweet potato cut into cubes

Method
1. Heat the olive oil in a saucepan or casserole.
2. Add in the sweet potato cubes and lightly brown it.
3. Add in the leek, ginger and carrots and cook for 3 minutes.
4. Stir in the turmeric and cumin powder and stir in for about 2 minutes.
5. Add in the vegetable or chicken broth and bring to a boil.
6. Once boiled, reduce to a simmer and cook for another 15 minutes till the chicken is tender.
7. Mash everything up with a soup blender.
8. Remove from heat and let the soup cool for 10 minutes before consumption.
9. Keep the remaining soup in a separate container in the fridge for consumption within the next 2 days.

3. Sweet pea soup with fresh mint

Green peas are a nutrient powerhouse and they contain a high dose of phytonutrients. They are rich in Vitamins A, B-1, B-2, B-3, B-6, C and vitamin K-1 for maintaining good bone health. Peas are also high in fiber and low in fat, a good source of vegetable protein. Green peas also contain high amounts of polyphenol called Coumestrol, which helps to prevent stomach cancer.

4-6 servings

Ingredients:
- 2 tbsp extra virgin olive oil
- 1/4 cup sliced white leeks
- 1/4 cup cubed zucchini
- 6 cups organic vegetable or chicken broth
- 1 Kg of frozen peas thawed
- 1/4 cup organic coconut milk
- 1/3 cup fresh mint leaves
- sea salt and pepper for taste

Method
1. Heat the oil in a saucepan or a casserole over medium heat.
2. Add in the leek and zucchini and cook till slightly softened for about 3 minutes.
3. Add in the broth and the peas and bring to a boil.
4. Remove from heat and bring it to a simmer for 15 minutes.
5. Use a soup blender and blend everything till it becomes a thick soup.
6. Remove from heat and let the soup cool for 10 minutes before consumption.
7. Keep the remaining soup in a separate container in the fridge for consumption within the next 2 days.

4. Sweet potato, kale, cauliflower and onions gratin

Kale is a superfood belonging to the cruciferous vegetable family with a wide range of phytonutrients and antioxidants. Kale is high in vitamin A, C and K, and contains natural sulfur compounds to enhance the sulfation process in detoxification with cancer-fighting properties. It is also a high source of fibre, which helps lower blood sugar and lower the risk of developing diabetes.

Ingredients

1. 1 sweet potato - sliced into thin rounds
2. 1 cauliflower head - chopped into small pieces
3. 1 bunch kale
4. 1 onion
5. 2 cloves garlic
6. 300ml organic coconut milk
7. 1 tbsp rosemary herb/mixed herbs
8. salt and pepper to taste

Method

1. Preheat oven to 180*C.
2. In a saucepan, put in 1 tbsp of olive oil and sauté the onions, garlic and chopped kale together until they are softened and slightly brown.
3. Grease a 9X9 inch baking pan and arrange the sweet potato slices in a single layer.
4. Spread the cauliflower florets in an even manner over the sweet potatoes.
5. Spread the kale mixture over the cauliflower mixture.
6. Whisk together the organic coconut milk, salt, pepper, nutmeg and rosemary/mixed herbs. Pour the mixture over the vegetables in a baking dish.
7. Place the dish in the oven and bake for 40min at 180*C until the potatoes are cooked through and the sauce is bubbling.
8. Remove from the oven and allow to cool 10 minutes before serving.

5. Black bean burger with cashews and carrots

Makes 6 burgers servings

Ingredients
- 1 large celery
- 1 medium carrot peeled and shredded
- 1/4 cup roasted cashews
- 2cups cooked or canned black beans
- 1/3 cup steel-cut oats
- 1 1/2 tsp vegetable bouillon powder
- 1 tsp ground cumin
- 1 tsp balsamic vinegar
- 1 tsp extra virgin olive oil
- 1 egg, beaten

Method
1. Put the celery, carrot and cashews in a food processor. Pulse to chop coarsest.
2. Add the beans, oats, bouillon powder, cumin, vinegar and 1 tbsp olive oil. Pulse until mixed evenly.
3. Cover and refrigerate for 1 hour or overnight.
4. Form the bean patties into 6 patties. Coat the patties with egg wash.
5. Heat the olive oil in a pan over medium heat.
6. Sautéed the patties until lightly brown - about 3 minutes on each side. Alternatively, bake in oven at 180*C for about 20 minutes.
7. Cool the patties for about 3 minutes before serving.
8. Put the patties between spelt burgers with a few slices of avocado to serve.

6. Lentil and pumpkin soup

Pumpkins are a high source of fibre, which is also packaged with vitamins and minerals while relatively low in calories. In addition, they contain antioxidants such as alpha-carotene, beta-carotene and beta-cryptoxanthin, which helps to remove free radicals from our body. It is also very high in beta-carotene, a carotenoid that turns into vitamin A in the body.

Servings: 4

Ingredients
- 750gm pumpkin (alternatively use sweet potatoes)
- 2 tbsp olive oil
- 1 onion peeled and finely chopped
- 1 cup of zucchini finely chopped
- 1/2 cup of lentils
- 1L water or organic chicken or vegetable broth
- 1 tsp paprika/cayenne pepper
- 1tbsp finely chopped parsley to garnish
- salt and pepper to taste

Method
1. In a saucepan, heat the olive oil in medium heat and fry the onions till brown. Add in the zucchini and sauté them in the saucepan for about 2 minutes.
2. Add in the lentil and the paprika/cayenne pepper and stir well.
3. Add in the pumpkin cubes and stir for about 2-3 minutes.
4. Add in the water or vegetable or chicken broth and bring it to a boil.
5. Then simmer on low heat for about 15 minutes till the lentil and pumpkin are soft.
6. Blitz the soup with a soup blender into a purée state.
7. Add salt and pepper to taste.
8. Add chopped parsley for garnish.

7. Asian Sesame Slaw

The Asian sesame slaw salad is rich in phytonutrients from all the colorful vegetables with the added goodness of good fatty acids from whole cashews, sesame seeds and fiber from the quinoa.

Ingredients:
- 3 cups of red cabbage, shredded
- 3 cups of green cabbage, shredded
- 1 cup of grated carrot
- 1 bunch fresh cilantro
- 4 tbsp green onions, diced
- 1 1/2 cup cooked quinoa
- 1 tbsp toasted black/white sesame seeds
- 1/3 cup whole cashews toasted and chopped

For the dressing:
- 2 cloves garlic, minced
- 2 tsp fresh grated ginger
- 2 tsp stevia
- 3 tbsp rice vinegar
- 1 tsp soy sauce
- 4 tbsp extra virgin olive oil
- 2 tbsp sesame oil
- 2 tsp squeezed lime juice

Method:
1. Cook the quinoa.
2. Heat up the pan and lightly toast the sesame seeds and cashews and remove from pan.
3. Mix the dressing ingredients in a small bowl.
4. In a large bowl, mix the cabbage, carrots, cilantro, green onions, black sesame seeds and cashews and mix thoroughly.
5. Add the dressing and the toasted sesame and nuts into the large mixing bowl.
6. Cool in the fridge for 10 minutes, then serve.

8. Healthy chicken soup with lentils

Chicken soup made from bone broth is very healing for the gut. Lentils belong to the legume family and are high in protein, polyphenols and are a good source of iron. They are also high in folate and magnesium and are a good source of fiber to add to the diet.

Servings 2-4

Ingredients:

- 2 large chicken drumsticks/thighs
- 1 large yellow onion finely chopped
- 1 tsp dried thyme
- 1 bay leaf
- 200gm green lentil (washed and soaked)
- 1-2 tbsp lemon juice
- 1 medium carrot peeled and finely chopped
- salt and pepper to taste

Method

1. In a saucepan, heat up the olive oil over medium heat. Fry the onions till slightly brown, then add the chicken and sauté till slightly brown.
2. Add the carrots and cook until slightly charred and set aside.
3. In a large saucepan, add the onions, chicken, carrots, thyme, bay leaf, parsley and cover with water. Bring to a boil. Turn down the heat to a simmer for about half an hour.
4. After half an hour, add the lentils into the pot and continue to simmer till soft for about 15-20min. Add more water as necessary.
5. When the chicken is soft, remove it from the pot and shred the meat. Add the shredded chicken back into the pot.
6. Add salt and pepper and some lemon juice to taste.

9. Pecan crusted catfish with pineapple slaw

Servings: 6

Ingredients
- 3/4 cup pecan nuts
- 1/4 cup breadcrumbs
- 1/2 tsp paprika powder
- 2 tbsp olive oil
- sea salt and pepper
- 3 catfish fillets (or salmon fillets)

For pineapple slaw
- 1/2 small green cabbage
- 1 cup pineapple chunks
- 2 tbsp rice vinegar
- 1 tbsp extra virgin olive oil
- sea salt and pepper for taste
- 1 medium carrot, peeled and finely shredded

Method
1. Preheat oven to 180*C.
2. Place the pecan nuts on a baking sheet and bake at 180*C for 5-10 minutes until lightly brown. Remove and cool.
3. In a food processor, combine the pecans, breadcrumbs, paprika powder and some sea salt and processed till finely chopped.
4. On a baking sheet, place the fillets onto the baking sheet, drizzle with olive oil and season with salt and pepper.
5. Dip the fillet onto the pecan mixture and coat both sides of the fish.
6. Bake the catfish for about 10 minutes in the oven until the fish is slightly brown on the outside.
7. Serve with the pineapple slaw on the side.

For the pineapple slaw
1. In a large bowl, add in the shredded cabbage, carrots and pineapple cubes, vinegar and extra virgin olive oil. Season with salt and pepper to taste.
2. Refrigerate in the fridge for about 30 minutes before servings.

10. Red lentil coconut curry with organic chicken

Coconut milk contains medium-chain triglycerides (MCTs), which stimulate energy production through thermogenesis and helps weight loss. Coconut milk also contains Lauric acid, which has antimicrobial and anti-inflammatory properties. However, coconut milk can be high in calories, so consume it in moderation.

Ingredients
- 1 tsp cumin seeds
- 1 tsp coriander seeds
- 1 tbsp coconut oil or grapeseed oil
- 1 yellow onion finely chopped
- 4 cloves garlic minced
- 1 tsp grated fresh ginger
- 3 red or green chilies chopped
- 400g chicken breast cut into cube size
- 1 tsp turmeric powder
- 1/4 tsp chili powder
- 1 cup of chopped tomatoes
- 1/2 cup of red lentils
- 500ml coconut milk
- fresh parsley finely chopped

Method
1. Add the cumin and coriander seeds to a saucepan and toast for 2 minutes under medium heat.
2. Add in the oil and the onions and cook till lightly brown.
3. Add in the garlic, ginger, green/red chilies and chicken pieces. Cook for 3 minutes till the chicken pieces are brown on the outside.
4. Add the chili powder, turmeric powder, chopped tomatoes and 500ml coconut milk.
5. Bring to a boil, then reduce heat to a simmer for about 15 minutes, stir regularly.
6. Add in the lentils and simmer for another 15 minutes until the lentils are soft and cooked.
7. Garnish with chopped parsley and serve.

You can freeze the above in a container and reheat until piping hot to be consumed the next day.

Final Thoughts

Our body is like a philharmonic orchestra. If one instrument is out of tune, the rest of the orchestra suffers as the music will not be soothing to the ears. Having toxins in our body is like having an instrument that goes out of tune. Unless we remove and sort out the toxins in the body, it will put an obstacle in our body and prevent our hormones and organs from working optimally. I have seen many patients who have suffered from chronic health issues like Hashimoto's thyroid disease or hypoadrenalism and chronic fatigue. Each patient is unique, and every symptom must be addressed individually. For a patient that suffers from multiple health problems, I would recommend the 3-pillar approach:

1. Remove the body of toxins
2. Replenish the gut and nutrients that the body is deficient in
3. Rebalance the hormones and optimize the cells

To face the truth, our world is getting more polluted and we are facing the dire consequences of having more toxins entering our food chain. Humanity is facing more health problems due to environmental toxins challenging our body's immune system. That is why diseases like Celiac disease and Hashimoto's are rising exponentially. In the past, our ancestors don't have to think much about detoxification as the food and water they drink don't harbor as much toxins as we do now. In this coming age, we have to incorporate detoxification strategies daily in our lives so as to prevent toxins from accumulating in our bodies and causing dire consequences to our health. I hope for this book to serve as a guide to you to understand some basic principles of detoxification and incorporate these practices more frequently in your life. As the saying goes, "Prevention is better than cure".

If you have any questions regarding detoxification or contents of this book related to toxins, do leave a short review for this book on Amazon and I would be happy to answer your question. You can contact me by subscribing to my website www.functionaldrhoseeyunn.com or simply follow me or send me a message via my instagram account @functionaldrhoseeyunn and I would be happy to get back to you regarding your question. If you have enjoyed the content of this book or find it beneficial in your own healing journey, please kindly leave a positive review for this book.

References

1. Chen, S. et al. "The Effect of Pollution on Migration : Evidence from China ." (2017).

2. The Health Effects Institute, the Institute for Health Metrics and Evaluation at the University of Washington, and the University of British Columbia., 2017. The State of Global Air 2017, The Health Effects Institute. (https://www.stateofglobalair.org/sites/default/files/SOGA2017_report.pdf)

3. Brown RC, Lockwood AH, Sonawane BR. Neurodegenerative diseases: An overview of environmental risk factors. Environ Health Perspectives. 2005; 113: 1250-1256.

4. Hinkle PM, Kinsella PA. Cadmium uptake and toxicity via voltage sensitive calcium channels. J biol Chem. 1987; 262: 16333 - 16337.

5. Rap KSJ, Rao RV. Trace elements in Alzheimer's disease brain: a new hypothesis. All Rep. 1999; 2:241-246.

6. Hedge ML, Shanmgavelu P. Serum trace element levels and the complexity of inter-element relations in patients with Parkinson's disease. J Trace Elem Med Biol. 2004; 18:163-171.

7. Abelsohn AR, Sanborn M. Lead and children: clinical management for family physicians. Can Fam Physician. 2010;56(6):531-535.

8. Can L, Li XK, Song Y Essentiality, toxicology and chelation therapy of zinc and copper. Curr <Med Chem. 2005; 12:2753 - 63

9. Cornett CR, Markesbury WR, Emmanuel WD. (1998). Imbalances of trace elements related to oxidative damage in Alzheimer's disease brain. Neurotoxicity. 19:339 - 346.

10. Fukushima T. Tan X. Kanda H. Neuroepidemiology 2010; 34:18-24.

11. Orisakwe OE. The role of lead and cadmium in psychiatry. N Am J Med Sci. 2014;6(8):370–376. doi:10.4103/1947-2714.139283

12. Vouldoukis I, Lacan D, Kamate C, et al. Antioxidant and anti-inflammatory properties of a Cucumis melo LC. extract rich in superoxide dismutase activity. J Ethnopharmacol. 2004 Sep;94(1):67-75.

13. Senile hair graying: H2O2 mediated oxidative stress affects human hair color by blunting methionine sulfoxide repair. J. M. Wood H. Decker H. Hartmann B. Chavan H. Rokos J. D. Spencer S. Hasse M. J. Thornton M. Shalbaf R. Paus K. U. Schallreuter

14. Agency for Toxic Substances and Disease Registry (ATSDR. Public Health Service. Atlanta: U.S. Department of Health and Human Services; 1999. Toxicological Profile for Lead.

15. Agency for Toxic Substances and Disease Registry (ATSDR) Case Studies in Environmental Medicine - Lead Toxicity. Atlanta: Public Health Service, U.S. Department of Health and Human Services; 1992.

16. JAMA.2013;309(12):1241-1250

17. Comparison of Chelating Agents DMPS, DMSA, and EDTA for the diagnosis and treatment of chronic metal exposure. British Journal of Medicine and Medical Research 4(9):1821-1835, 2014

18. https://www.hchcares.org/wp-content/uploads/2016/09/Detox_Food_Plan_Comprehensive_Guide.pdf

19. Olszewer Z, Carter JP. "EDTA Chelation Therapy: A Retrospective Study of 2,870 Patients," Journal of Advancement in Medicine 2, nos. 1&2 (1989): 197 - 213

20. Olsezewer E, Sabbag FC, Carter P. "A Pilot Double Blind Study of Sodium-Magnesium EDTA in Peripheral Vascular Disease," JNatl Med Assn 82, no.3 (1990): 174-77

21. Lamas GA, Goertz C, Boineau R, Mark DB, Rozema T, Nahin RL, Drisko JA, Lee KL. Design of the Trial to Assess Chelation Therapy (TACT). Am Heart J. 2012 Jan;163(1):7-12. doi: 10.1016/j.ahj.2011.10.002. PMID: 22172430; PMCID: PMC3243954.

22. California Posion Control System. Antidote chart 2012. Available at: http://www.calpoison.org/hcp/CPCS_antidote_chart.pdf